THE COMPLETE GUIDE TO

EXERCISING AWAY STRESS

Other titles in **THE COMPLETE GUIDE** series

*The Complete Guide to
Circuit Training
by Debbie Lawrence, Bob Hope*

*The Complete Guide to
Postnatal Fitness
by Judy DiFiore*

*The Complete Guide to
Endurance Training
by Jon Ackland*

*The Complete Guide to
Strength Training
by Anita Bean*

*The Complete Guide to
Exercise in Water
by Debbie Lawrence*

*The Complete Guide to
Stretching
by Christopher Norris*

*The Complete Guide to
Core Stability
by Matt Lawrence*

*The Complete Guide to
Sports Massage
by Tim Paine*

*The Complete Guide to
Studio Cycling
by Rick Kiddle*

*The Complete Guide to
Sports Nutrition
by Anita Bean*

*The Complete Guide to
Exercise to Music
by Debbie Lawrence*

*The Complete Guide to
Sports Motivation
by Ken Hodge*

THE **COMPLETE GUIDE TO**

Debbie Lawrence

EXERCISING AWAY STRESS

A & C Black • London

Note

While every effort has been made to ensure that the content of this book is as technically accurate and as sound as possible, neither the author nor the publisher can accept responsibility for any injury or loss sustained as a result of the use of this material

Published in 2005 by A & C Black (Publishers) Ltd
37 Soho Square, London W1D 3QZ
www.acblack.com

Copyright © 2005 by Debbie Lawrence

ISBN 0 7136 7240 4

A CIP catalogue record for this book is available from the British Library.

A & C Black uses paper produced with elemental chlorine-free pulp, harvested from managed sustainable forests.

Acknowledgements
Cover photograph © Jump
Illustrations by Jean Ashley

Typeset in 10½ on 12pt Baskerville BE Regular by Palimpsest Book Production Limited, Polmont, Stirlingshire

Printed and bound in Great Britain by
Biddles Ltd., King's Lynn

CONTENTS

ACKNOWLEDGEMENTS

Writing the acknowledgements is always my favourite part and brings a huge smile to my face. Writing is one of my greatest passions. It is food for my soul and what my heart truly loves doing.

The subject nature of this book tempts me to thank all the situations and people who have contributed to my feeling stressed, for without those experiences I certainly would not have learned to understand and manage my own stress, let alone produce a book for others to use as a resource to help them manage theirs.

Let it be known that, despite my experiences of stress, I am still not a master in managing stress, pretty much, I teach what I most have to learn and I am continuously learning.

As always I have lots of people I would like to thank for their contribution to my life:

My really special girly pals – Alex Carr, Sheena Land, Janet Forster, Clare Framp – for all the special things you bring. Thanks also to Clare for contributing to the section on Pilates.

My great friend Qaalfa Dibeehi, an inspirational man who has taught me a lot.

My lovely friends and fellow students on the Inter-psyche Diploma of Integrative Psychotherapy and Counselling, with particular thanks and much love to Sue Goode (whom I need to thank for her fabulous contribution to the section on creativity); Margaret Tanton (a great youth worker); Bobbie Akhurst (a fabulous person and mother); Mike the Bike (for his childlike sense of humour and being a storyteller); Virginia Maclane (for embracing her feelings); and Lynn Phipps (for being loving and also for the humorous texts).

Very special thanks to Sheila Norris, my therapist: for providing the most wonderful environment for me to explore myself and experience my deepest emotions safely and without judgement.

My lecturers at Inter-psyche who have all inspired me greatly with their very unique and special styles: Mike Berry, Graz Kowzsun, Anup and Brenda; my supervisor at Inter-psyche – Christine Roeder (for appreciating what I refer to as my 'airy-fairy' approach?); my therapy and personal training clients from whom I always continue to learn.

Thank you also to Julia Stanton and Claire Dunn of A & C Black for getting this project off the ground!

Writing this book has been my pleasure and my stress ☺

Debbie Lawrence

INTRODUCTION

Stress is a recognised threat to our mental health and overall well-being. Stress-related disorders are listed on the ICD – 10 mental health classification system for mental disorders. These include: anxiety disorders, phobias, obsessive-compulsive and post-traumatic stress disorders. The mental health foundation suggests that twelve million adults visit their GP each year with mental health problems. Most of these are diagnosed as suffering from anxiety and depression that is **stress-related.**

Stress is recognised as a major cause of absenteeism from work (HMSO, 1988). Occupational stress has been identified as a major health and safety issue in British workplaces (TUC, 1996) and the prescription of psychotherapeutic drugs has increased over recent years. Stress has also been linked as a contributory factor to a number of other medical conditions, including coronary heart disease, hypertension, strokes, some cancers, irritable bowel syndrome and so on.

From the moment we are born to the moment of our death we are exposed to experiences and life events that can have either a positive or negative affect on our mental and emotional well-being. Work (promotion, redundancy), relationships (marriage, divorce, arguments), life-changing events (births, deaths), family matters (health, vacations) and financial pressures (mortgages, loans) are all common causes of stress that will affect most people at some stage in their life. Therefore, it appears that stress is becoming a **natural part** of modern living.

If stress is to be viewed as a naturally occurring response to **living in a fast-paced world**, then managing stress and coping skills for stressful situations must also be seen as a priority. **Training and education** on how to manage stress need to be provided if individuals are to live happily, peacefully and in harmony with themselves and each other.

Personal trainers frequently act as sounding boards for their clients' problems. They can also play a key role within a stress management programme by recommending exercise and activity and promoting behavioural changes that will help to manage the physical demands of stress. They can also act as a resource for providing information on other practical techniques that will assist with the emotional, mental and behavioural effects of stress. However, personal trainers need to be aware of the limitations of their knowledge and also of their personal boundaries. They need to be able to recognise when it may benefit an individual to be referred to other specialists such as counsellors, psychotherapists or alternative therapists. Alternative therapies (massage, reiki and so on) can also play an important role if an individual appears particularly overwhelmed by their stresses.

The aim of this book is to provide a resource for all persons interested in stress and stress management techniques. There is a broad range of knowledge available about this subject area. In this book, I have attempted to introduce fields that can be explored and researched further by interested persons, through professional training and qualifications.

I have drawn the information from my personal experience and my work experience as a personal trainer, a counsellor and a teacher. I have also drawn from my personal study of these areas of expertise to put together this guide.

Part One attempts to provide a definition of stress and explores possible causes of stress and how perception and resources will influence our ability to cope and keep stress levels to a healthy, balanced level. It also explores the signs and symptoms of stress and describes how our bodies respond immediately in stressful situations and how longer-term exposure to stress can impact our health and well-being. The final chapter in this section explores the benefits of exercise and how exercise can help to manage stress.

Part Two outlines a number of strategies and practical techniques and exercises that can be used to assist with managing the physical, behavioural, mental and emotional signs and symptoms of stress. These techniques can be used to assist with both personal stress management and the management of our clients' stress. Some examples of specific exercises and activities that can assist with stress management are also suggested.

Part Three describes a model for changing behaviour and identifies the strategies that can be used to promote positive movement through all stages of the change process. It also identifies some of the skills and qualities that will enable personal trainers and fitness instructors to assist clients to manage stress.

Part Four explores specific case studies and describes the specific strategies and exercises they have selected to help them manage their stress.

It is hoped that this book will be used as a resource that contributes to making life a happier, healthier and more peaceful experience for more individuals.

> 'Even a happy life cannot be without a measure of darkness, and the word "happiness" would lose its meaning if it were not balanced by sadness'
>
> *Carl Jung*

> 'A crisis event often explodes the illusions that anchor our lives'
>
> *Robert Veninga*

ALL ABOUT STRESS

PART **ONE**

This section of the book provides some basic information about stress. It moves towards attempting to find a definition of stress and explores possible causes of stress and how perception and resources will influence our ability to cope and keep stress levels to a healthy, balanced level.

It also explores the mental, emotional, behavioural and physical signs and symptoms of stress and describes how our body responds immediately in stressful situations and how longer-term exposure to stress can impact our health and well-being.

The benefits of exercise and the role it plays in stress management are also explored.

The information in this section provides the groundwork for the subject matter in the rest of the book, which explores different strategies for managing or possibly exercising away stress.

WHAT IS STRESS?

What is stress?

Stress is not an easy thing to define; as a starting point, it can be viewed as a *psychological condition* that influences how we respond to life events and living. Life and living provide us with stimuli, which will be referred to as *stressors*. Each life stressor will place a *demand* on our internal and external coping *resources*. If the demands exceed our coping resources we will experience *negative* stress; if we are able to manage and utilise our resources to handle the situation we will experience *positive* stress.

A secondary point towards defining stress is that it can be viewed both *positively* and *negatively*, with the majority of people being more inclined to associate with the negative aspects of stress and define it as a negative experience rather than associating with it as a positive experience. Table 1.1 lists some of the negative and positive words people associate with stress.

The key thing to recognise is that if it is viewed positively stress or stressful situations can be *life-enhancing and enriching, and can encourage personal growth*. However, if it is viewed negatively it can be *life-destroying* and may lead to various physical and mental illnesses, poor performance at work, accidents, relationship problems and, ultimately, death.

Why do people view stress and situations differently?

Although it may seem obvious, it is important to recognise that people are different, they are born to different families in different cultures

Table 1.1	The negative and positive associations negative stress

Negative:

Anxiety pressure strain tension panic fear discomfort loss of control anger loss of power loss of hope overload effort burden troubles worry pain grief depression anger frustration distress failure no disappointment sadness boredom tiredness

Positive:

Challenge excitement stimulation power drive control hopeful enthusiasm adventure enjoyment fun happiness pleasure success achievement encouragement yes enjoyment reward satisfaction contentment creativity expression energy

with different social, educational and financial backgrounds and each has her or his own unique experience of life. They will therefore respond to life events differently and have their own unique *perceptions* about their circumstances and ability to meet life's demands and challenges. What one person perceives as a negatively stressful experience, another person may perceive as a positively stressful experience. A third point towards defining stress is that it is influenced by an individual's *perception*. A key thing to bear in mind here is that there is no right or wrong about these perceptions, just that they are unique to the individual.

Table 1.2	Example activity: How stressful would you find each of these experiences?										
How stressful would you find:	0 No Problem	1	2	3	4	5	6	7	8	9	10 Distress- ing
A bungee jump											
Speaking to a large audience of people											
Walking into a restaurant alone											
Winning a big prize on the lottery											
Being stood up on a date											
Going to an exercise class											
Picking up a spider											
Starting a new business											
Going on a first date											
Losing a lot of money											
Travelling abroad											
Starting a new relationship											
Confrontation											
Using the free weights area at a gym											
Ending a relationship											
Riding a bicycle											
Illness											
Getting a mortgage on a house											
Losing your job											
Discovering you are pregnant (females!)											
Being made redundant											
Starting a college course											
Taking an exam											
Teaching an aerobics class											
Getting married											
Passing an exam											

To explore your own perception of stress, use the example activity in Table 1.2. Grade each example on a scale of 0 (exciting/great/positive) to 10 (distressing/awful/negative). Try the exercise with a group of friends to explore how they perceive the different activities.

Why does perception affect stress?

Individuals' perceptions will depend on how they feel about the demands of a situation in relation to their awareness of the resources they feel they have to manage the situation. This will obviously affect how they respond to stressful

Table 1.3	Life experiences, prejudices and what we may experience mentally and emotionally
Life stresses we encounter	Birth, potty training, teething, infant school, controlling bodily functions, making friends, Sunday school, learning to walk and talk, parental divorce, school, acne, getting drunk, smoking, adolescence, sex, sexuality, dyslexia, wearing glasses, exams, driving test, first car, first relationship, first sexual experience, leaving home, income, responsibility, falling in love, heartbreak, living with someone, engagement, taking drugs, alcohol, stopping taking drugs, smoking, stopping smoking, abortion, miscarriage, losing job, being fired, death of family member/friend, crime, being a victim of crime, breakdown, university, jobs, house buying, moving house, marriage, infidelity, change of career, financial commitments, war, debts, holidays, taxes, mid-life crises, relationships ending, hobbies, travelling, new relationship, redundancy, family feuds, serious illness, family, pregnancy, giving birth, children, divorce, menopause, illness, retirement, bus pass, pension, old people's home, loss of independence, dying
Prejudices we experience	Language, age, money, gender, class, nationality, race, size, sexuality, physical ability, mental ability, religion, education, culture, language, accent, hair colour, postcode, social background, image, career, social group, salary, politics, morality, being beautiful, being ugly, intelligence, appearance
Messages we may hear	Be good, be perfect, be strong, not good enough, not wanted, not loved, not valued
Feelings we experience and behaviours they manifest	Depressed, lost, motivated to change, alcoholic, drug-dependent, angry, stressed, hurt, lonely, confused, desperate, unhappy, scared, misunderstood, insecure, pitiful, patronised, ridiculed, helpless, resentful, isolated, embarrassed, flattered, honoured, different, motivated, losing confidence, determination, aggressive, empowered, strong, vulnerable, low in self-esteem, happy, contented, satisfied, elated, stupid, dizzy, high, nervous, moody, excited, complacent, suicidal, fearful, inspired, worthless, melancholic, wiser, disgusted, frustrated, high in self esteem, bitter, confident, rejected, alone, humiliated

events. Therefore, a fourth point towards defining stress is that there needs to be a balance between the *perceived demands* of a task or situation and the *coping resources* the person believes they have to manage the task or situation for them to respond healthily. Life brings many experiences and our response to and support through these transition phases can have an impact on how we respond in stressful situations throughout life. Table 1.3 outlines some of the average life experiences, prejudices we experience, messages we hear (which can be external or internal talk) and the feelings evoked.

Any task, situation or life event has the potential to become negatively stressful if it is perceived as being more than the person is able to cope with at that moment in time with the resources they perceive they have available. This will throw our stress levels out of balance. The way we move through our life experiences and the support we find along the way (from friends, family and significant others) can affect how we manage stress throughout our lives.

Recommended reading regarding some of the psychological theories on how people grow and develop is provided at the end of this book.

Some people have many resources but may believe they are unable to cope, whereas other people have fewer resources but believe they are able to manage the demands upon them. Table 1.4 illustrates a range of potential demands and a range of potential resources. From this perspective, a person's belief system about themselves and their ability to cope – their *self-efficacy* – may provide a fifth point in defining stress. For persons with a low self-efficacy, a supportive relationship that helps them to identify and utilise the internal and external resources they have accessible will be most effective in helping them increase awareness and overcome their stressors. This is probably best achieved by a short-term therapeutic intervention such as counselling and psychotherapy or, possibly, a self-help book. Information regarding other support services is also provided at the end of this book.

The number of potential stressors one has in one's life at any one time can also affect the stress

Table 1.4	Potential demands and resources
Potential demands may arise from:	*Potential resources may come from:*
Work	Mental attitude, aptitude, knowledge, mental health, self-discipline, self-esteem and self-efficacy (belief in one's ability)
Relationships	
Family	Emotional intelligence, self-awareness and assertiveness
Home	Physical fitness, skills and ability
Holidays	Medical health and wellness
Study courses	Social support systems
Starting an exercise programme	Nutritional and dietary balance
Financial circumstances	Spiritual beliefs (belief in a higher power or alternative religious beliefs)
All of the above	Financial sources

NB: The effects of these demands and resources on specific case studies will be explored throughout the book.

balance. A comparatively small stressor may be enough to tip the balance to an unhealthy level for a person with a large number of other stressors in his or her life. Table 1.5 illustrates how stress levels can move out of balance.

Alternatively, a person with insufficient stressors may also experience stress negatively and unhealthily. Their resources will be under-challenged and under-stimulated, leading to feelings of boredom and lifelessness. The key appears to be for each individual to find the right balance between demands and resources for her- or himself. This will be different for each person.

Stress is an inevitable part of living. We need some stress to function healthily. The key is to maintain a healthy balance by:

- managing the demands made upon us; and
- building our coping resources.

Specific exercises and strategies to manage stress and stressful situations will be explored in Part Two. As an introduction to managing stress we can use the principles of training for physical fitness. The difference would be in its application, the aim being to reduce rather than increase the principles. Table 1.6 describes the principles of training applied to managing stress.

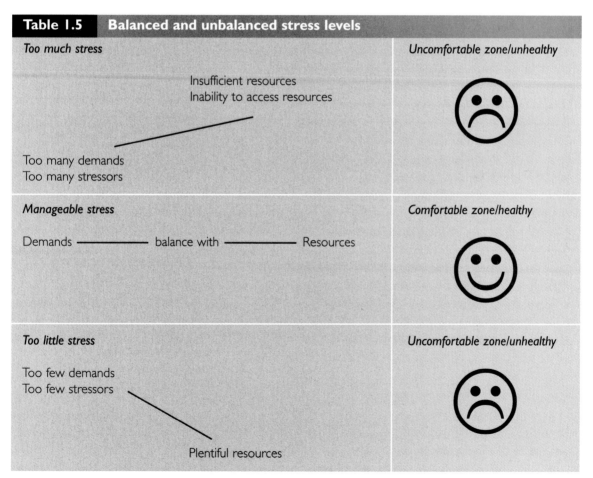

| Table 1.5 | Balanced and unbalanced stress levels |

Too much stress

Insufficient resources
Inability to access resources

Too many demands
Too many stressors

Uncomfortable zone/unhealthy

Manageable stress

Demands ———— balance with ———— Resources

Comfortable zone/healthy

Too little stress

Too few demands
Too few stressors

Plentiful resources

Uncomfortable zone/unhealthy

Table 1.6	The fitness training principles applied to managing too much stress
Frequency	How often are we being subjected to specific stressors?
	What strategies are available to change the frequency?
Intensity	
Repetition	How many stressors are there?
Resistance	Are the stressors large or small?
Rest	Are we able to take a break from the stressors?
Range	Are we able to remove any of the stressors, delegate and prioritise demands?
Time	How long will each of the stressors be in place?
	Is there a light at the end of the tunnel?
Type	What type of stressors? Positive or negative?
	How is each stressor affecting us (mentally, emotionally, physically, behaviourally)
	Which of the stressors are changeable?
Adherence	What resources do we have to manage the stressors?
	Do we need different resources for different stressors?
	What additional resources are accessible?

Chapter summary

To summarise the points raised in this chapter:

- Stress can be defined as a psychological condition.
- It can be viewed positively (which is healthy) or negatively (which is unhealthy).
- It will be influenced by an individual's perception of her or his life and environment.
- It will be influenced by the perceived demands being placed on the person from the environment and the perceived resources he or she has available.
- It will be influenced by a person's belief in her or his own ability to cope.
- To keep stress at a healthy level we need to balance the frequency, intensity, time and type of demands made upon us and build our coping resources.

And to conclude this chapter – the serenity prayer read from the lighter and darker aspects of the personality:

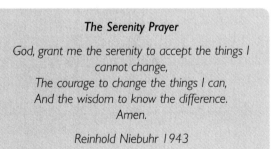

The Serenity Prayer

God, grant me the serenity to accept the things I cannot change,
The courage to change the things I can,
And the wisdom to know the difference.
Amen.

Reinhold Niebuhr 1943

The Alternative Serenity Prayer

Grant me the serenity to accept the things I
cannot change,
The courage to change the things I cannot accept,
And the wisdom to hide the bodies of those I had to
kill today because they irritated me.
And also, help me to remember that the toes I step
on today may be connected to the feet I have to kiss
tomorrow.

Help me to give 100 per cent at work:
12 per cent on Monday
23 per cent on Tuesday
40 per cent on Wednesday
20 per cent on Thursday and
5 per cent on Friday.

And help me to remember, when I feel real low and
I'm having a bad day and people are trying to wind
me up that it takes:
48 muscles to frown
28 muscles to smile and only 4 to extend my arm
and punch them in the jaw!

Author unknown

THE PHYSIOLOGY OF STRESS

2

Having gathered some basic information from the last chapter on what stress is, this chapter moves on to explore how stress can have an effect on our overall well-being. It also looks at the stress response, of which a basic knowledge is needed to understand why certain stress management interventions can be effective.

What are the effects of unhealthy stress?

Stress can manifest in a number of ways. It is often when we experience an *accumulation* of the different signs and symptoms that we stop, take notice, become aware of our stress and make steps towards finding solutions. Table 2.1 provides an example of some of the signs and symptoms of stress.

Awareness of how stress manifests in ourselves and others will assist with the stress management process and help to find appropriate strategies to manage the stressors.

How do our bodies respond physiologically in times of stress?

While evolution has provided us with many developments to human physiology, the way we respond in stressful situations is rather more primitive and comparatively less evolved. In the days when we lived in caves and had to hunt for our food and fight off or run from wild beasts, the 'fight or flight' response was a great asset. In emergency situations that we experience today (for example, a fire) the triggering of this response is useful to assist our physical escape. Table 2.2 outlines how the different systems of the body respond to stressful situations. Note: The stress response 'fight or flight' is a complex response that is explored in greater depth in related texts, some of which are listed as further reading.

The key issue is that most of the stressors we experience in modern life are less physical in nature, yet our bodies still respond in the old, primitive way and prepare us for action to either fight or flee (see case study 1 overleaf). With this in mind, and the awareness that a great proportion of the public is not achieving healthy targets of physical activity, stress can accumulate and build up in the body. This is one of the reasons why increasing physical activity and exercise are so beneficial for managing some of the signs and symptoms of stress.

In addition, there is great power in recognising that the monster stressor we perceive is frequently not as life-threatening as we may initially think. In many instances, if we are able to step back from the situation and gather our perspective, we can find a variety of creative new ways to handle the situation and minimise the size of the stressor. Strategies and exercises for dealing with the various signs and symptoms of stress will be explored further in Part Two.

Table 2.1	Signs and symptoms of unhealthy stress		
Physical	*Mental*	*Emotional*	*Behavioural*
Spots	Irrational thoughts	Sadness	Eating more or less
Shoulder tension	Mental fatigue	Depression	Drinking more stimulants
Skin disorders	Poor decision-making	Anger	Smoking more
Chest pain	Low self-esteem	Fear	Swearing
Increased heart rate	Low self-worth	Panic	Aggression
Nervous indigestion	Inability to listen	Irritability	Violence
Fast, shallow breathing	Procrastination	Boredom	Crime
Upper back hunched	Excessive self-criticism	Loneliness	Crying
Yawning/sighing	Egocentricity	Jealousy	Increased or decreased sexual libido
Increased blood pressure	Accident proneness	Resentment	Excessive talking
Abdominal pain	Making more mistakes	Helplessness	Foot-tapping
Sexual difficulties	Negative outlook on life	Powerlessness	Inability to sit still
Clenched jaw	Blaming others or self	Insecurity	Picking at skin
Menstrual disorders	Judgementalism	Frustration	Grinding of teeth
Flatulence	Criticism of self and others	Tearfulness	Rapid eye movements
Allergies		Lethargy	Gripping hands
Hair loss		Lack of focus	Argumentative behaviour
Dry mouth		Anxiety	Nervous laughter
Tense forehead/ headaches		Loss of hope	Driving faster

Table 2.2	How the body responds to stress
Body system/part	**Response to stress**
The senses: • hearing • smell • sight • touch • taste • intuition	Pupils dilate to increase vision. All senses become more alert to respond to the perceived threat. Pain reactions are numbed as a method of protecting against physical danger.
The brain	The cerebral cortex evaluates information provided by the senses and decides on the response to be taken. The limbic system (the emotional brain) adds emotion, such as fear, anger, excitement etc. and adds to the decision made by the cerebral cortex. The hypothalamus receives the information from the cerebral cortex and limbic system and sends messages via the autonomic nervous system (parasympathetic and sympathetic) to the body organs and hormones are released.
The sympathetic nervous system	This system is the 'accelerator' system for the body. It plays a key role in preparing the body for fight or flight. The action of this system is brought about by the neurotransmitter noradrenaline, which will trigger the release of hormones from certain organs.
The parasympathetic nervous system	This system provides the 'braking' effect to different body systems. This action is brought about by a neurotransmitter called Acetylcholine. When we need to fight or flee this system becomes INACTIVE, which can be linked to other physical responses noted below. The role of this system is to save energy, assist digestion and protect against foreign bodies. Increased activity of this system would lead to the secretion of tears, saliva, mucus (from nose and throat) and gastric juice in the stomach. The system is brought into play when the brain receives the message that the stressful situation is over.
The hormonal system	The nervous system triggers the hormonal system to act on the organs of the body. The adrenal glands lie at the top of each kidney; they have an outer structure (the adrenal cortex) and an inner structure (the adrenal medulla). The adrenal medulla releases the hormones adrenaline and noradrenaline when we feel we need to fight or flee. If we feel more in control and ready to fight we display aggression and anger and the predominant hormone released is noradrenaline. This hormone also gives feelings of pleasure, excitement and arousal and stimulates the sensory organs. If we feel out of control and ready to run away, the predominant hormone is adrenaline. The effects of this hormone are less pleasurable; they are in response to fear and panic.

Table 2.2	How the body responds to stress cont.
Body system/part	*Response to stress*
The hormonal system cont.	Another hormone, cortisol, is released by the adrenal cortex both throughout and after the stressful event with the intention to reduce swelling and assist the healing of wounds received from physical danger. Cortisol also suppresses the body's allergic reaction to irritants such as dust, which could slow the body down when it needs to move. Cortisol plays a greater role in managing long-term stress. This is discussed later on in this chapter.
The heart	Starts to beat faster to increase the supply of blood and oxygen to specific body areas to create energy to fight or flee. Blood pressure will increase in response to the increase in heart beat.
The blood	Blood flows through the body faster in response to increased heart rate, blood pressure and vessel dilation. Clotting agents are released into the bloodstream to decrease bleeding in anticipation of physical harm.
The lungs	Adrenalin dilates the airways and breathing rate increases and becomes deeper, so that more oxygen can be taken in and carbon dioxide expelled.
The spleen	Is also stimulated by the sympathetic nervous system and releases more red blood cells so that more oxygen can be transported.
The liver	Glycogen and fat are released into the bloodstream and are transported to provide energy for the working muscles needed to fight or flee.
The muscles	Muscular capillaries dilate and more blood and oxygen flow into the muscles in preparation for creating energy to fight or flee. The muscles tense in preparation to fight or flee.
The skin	Blood is diverted away from the skin to reduce anticipated bleeding. Sweat is produced to keep the body cool.
The digestive system	Blood is diverted away from this system.
The sexual organs	Blood flow diverts away from these organs.

Stress and health: how do our bodies respond when we are exposed to stress for longer durations?

In times of longer-term stress, and when stressors persist, for example being out of work or managing relationships at work and at home, our bodies have to find additional ways of coping. In these times the pituitary gland and adrenal cortex system play a greater role to manage energy needs to meet the extra demands. Table 2.3 outlines some of the longer-term effects of stress.

Chapter summary

While stress is predominantly a condition of the mind, it is clear from the information provided in this chapter that the stress our mind perceives can have an impact on our physical health. The way we think will trigger certain physiological responses. This will in turn have an impact on our emotions and our behaviour. With this is mind, the techniques and exercises explored in Part Two are intended as a guide towards managing stress more holistically and healthily, as all systems are interlinked and need to work together in unity and balance. An imbalance in one area will cause an imbalance in other areas. My aim is to demonstrate that all areas are important and all need to be exercised.

Case study I

X is at work and her boss delegates a further workload to manage and be completed by a stated deadline. X has initial thoughts of all the other work she has and does not think she is able to cope; this leads to further thoughts about being unable to manage, which trigger fear of being seen as incompetent. X is already overloaded and this additional 'demand' pushes her over the edge of her comfort zone. She is consumed with this fear for the whole day. When she arrives home she is tired, tearful and irritable. From a physical perspective she would have triggered the responses listed in Table 2.2. The emotional response of fear would have caused the predominance of the hormone adrenaline to rise, which leads biologically to wanting to run away, which is how X described the event.

That evening X attends an exercise class, which releases some of the physical tension that has built up. She later telephones a friend to discuss the day and they end up laughing about the situation. The positive actions she takes in the evening help to combat some of the tension and emotion produced by the day's stress.

An alternative, proactive coping strategy to manage future scenarios:
X could assert herself and explain to her boss that she already has a large workload. She could suggest they negotiate an agreeable and workable time-frame for the work to be completed.

Table 2.3	Longer-term physical effects of stress
Long-term stress	*The effects on the body*
The hormonal system	The pituitary–adrenal cortex system is more dominant in times of long-term stress. Cortisol levels are increased to supply the energy to meet these increased demands. Excessive levels of cortisol suppress the immune system, which makes us more susceptible to illness and disease. This is perhaps one of the most important things to bear in mind as many diseases are linked with stress.
The immune system	Suppression of the immune system can make us more susceptible to colds and flu and other diseases that effect the immune system, such as some cancers. Long-term stress can also affect the body's healing and repair processes, which may have an impact on the health of our bones (leading possibly to osteoporosis) and tissues.
The sex hormones	The sex hormones increase when we are feeling more secure. Testosterone (and the female version, androstenedione) levels can increase when feelings of power, control, dominance and success are experienced in a particular situation. Levels of sex hormones can play a key role in influencing our social behaviour and relationships (support systems). Suppression of the reproductive system can lead to cessation of menstruation in women, impotence in men and loss of libido in both genders.
The respiratory system	Long-term stress triggers to the respiratory system may induce and increase the symptoms of asthma and other respiratory conditions.
The digestive system	Suppression of the digestive system may lead to diseases such as constipation, diarrhoea, irritable bowel and so on.
The heart and	Excess blood sugars may contribute to furring of the artery walls (atherosclerosis), which may lead to coronary artery disease.
Other systems circulatory system	Long-term stress can have an effect on managing blood sugar levels and may be linked to adult onset diabetes.

THE BENEFITS OF EXERCISE

3

Why is exercise important?

Physical fitness is one of the essential components of and contributors to our overall health and total fitness. Total fitness embraces working on the whole person and integrating medical fitness, nutritional fitness, social fitness, spiritual fitness, mental fitness and emotional fitness to maintain the individual's well-being. Some of these aspects are explored further in Part Two.

Long-term participation in a well-designed exercise programme can improve all the components that contribute to the physical fitness of an individual. The components that are most essential for maintaining our fitness for life and health are:

- cardiovascular fitness;
- muscular strength and endurance; and
- flexibility.

A further component that is needed additionally by sports people is motor fitness. They will need additional training of more specific skill-related components, which include: agility, balance, reaction time, speed, power and co-ordination.

In relation to stress management, awareness of the physiological 'fight or flight' stress response as described in the previous chapter can help us to recognise and understand how exercise in particular can have an immediate positive effect on managing stress.

This chapter explores the immediate benefits of exercise, discusses each of the components of physical fitness and identifies how exercise can contribute towards the longer-term and more holistic well-being of an individual.

What are the immediate benefits and effects of exercise?

When we start to exercise our heart rate and blood pressure increase and we begin to breathe faster and more deeply; our body temperature rises and our capillaries (small blood vessels) dilate, all of which allows more oxygen to be circulated around the body.

Our neuromuscular pathways are also activated, making us more attuned to our bodies and how they are moving. Our minds have to concentrate and focus on what we are doing. This can distract us from thinking about worries and hassles that have disturbed us through the day, providing a rest for the mind, which can promote greater mental awareness and alertness when we stop exercising.

In addition, our muscles have to contract and use sugars that may have built up through the day as a consequence of the stress response, providing an appropriate release. The movement of the joints and muscles can also provide release for any physical tension that has been created in our body and it becomes easier for our body to open up and move freely and more easily.

A further benefit is that when we are exercising we release feel-good hormones called endorphins. These create a positive feeling that can last much longer than the exercise session itself. Another benefit is that when we make time to exercise, we know it is doing us good, and it is uplifting to be taking positive action for looking after ourselves. Making time to exercise is an empowering action.

What is cardiovascular fitness?

Cardiovascular fitness is the ability of the heart, lungs and circulatory system to transport and utilise oxygen efficiently and remove waste products from the body. It is sometimes referred to as cardio-respiratory fitness, stamina, or aerobic fitness.

What are the long-term benefits of cardiovascular training?

We need a strong heart and efficient respiratory and circulatory systems to maintain our quality of life. A weak heart and inefficient respiratory and circulatory systems are more susceptible to diseases that can cause premature death. Coronary heart disease is the highest cause of death in the Western world and both stress and physical inactivity are recognised as contributing factors to this disease. Increased physical activity and improved cardiovascular fitness can assist in preventing us from contracting such diseases.

Regular, long-term participation in specific activities to build up physical fitness will improve the efficiency of the heart, lungs and blood vessels. The heart will become stronger, allowing it to pump a greater volume of blood with each contraction (stroke volume). The capillary network in our muscles will also expand, which allows the transportation of more oxygen to the body cells and the swifter removal of waste products. The size and number of mitochondria, the cells in which aerobic energy is produced, will also increase. This in turn will enable us to deliver and utilise the oxygen that our muscles receive more efficiently. Oxygen is essential for the long-term production of energy that keeps us alive.

Therefore, increasing our delivery of oxygen and removal of waste products will assist with performance of all activities.

Long-term cardiovascular training will also assist with managing cholesterol levels. The healthier cholesterol that helps clean the artery walls (High Density Lipoproteins – HDLs) will increase and the damaging cholesterol that furs and sticks to the artery walls (Low Density Lipoproteins – LDLs) will decrease. Cardiovascular training will also increase the metabolic rate, the rate at which we use energy or burn calories. If we perform these activities more frequently they can assist with weight management by potentially reducing our body fat and the lowering of cholesterol levels. The increased strength and efficiency of the cardiovascular system, coupled with the reduction in body fat and cholesterol levels, also potentially contributes to the normalising of elevated blood pressure. All these consequences have a positive effect on our health.

Summary of the long-term benefits of cardiovascular training

- Stronger heart muscle
- Increased stroke volume (amount of blood pumped with each contraction of the heart)
- Increased capillarisation (more blood vessels delivering blood and oxygen to the muscles)
- Increased mitochondria (cells in which aerobic energy is produced)
- Increased metabolic rate (rate at which we burn calories)
- Decreased body fat
- Healthier cholesterol balance (HDLs increase and LDLs decrease)
- Decreased blood pressure
- Decreased risk of coronary heart disease

How can we improve our cardiovascular fitness?

To improve cardiovascular fitness we need to perform rhythmical, continuous activities that use the larger muscles of the body. Some examples include:

- walking
- running
- cycling
- aerobic dancing
- line dancing
- rowing
- swimming.

These need to be performed on a regular basis, ideally between three and five times per week; at a moderate intensity to create a feeling of mild breathlessness without any unnecessary discomfort; and sustained for a prolonged duration, ideally between 20 and 30 minutes. Adherence to this type of exercise programme will do much to induce the long-term health improvements listed above. The recommended training requirements for improvements of cardiovascular fitness are outlined in table 3.1.

What is flexibility?

Flexibility is the ability of our joints and muscles to move through their full potential range of movement. It is sometimes referred to as suppleness or mobility.

Table 3.1	The recommended training requirements for improvements of cardiovascular fitness.
Frequency How often should we perform these activities?	Between 3 and 5 times a week. Ideally, we should vary the activities we perform and alter the impact to avoid repetitive strain or injury to the muscles and joints.
Intensity How hard should we be working?	Working at an intensity that causes the heart rate to elevate into the training zone (55–90 per cent) of maximum heart rate is sufficient, lower levels of intensity being appropriate for less active populations.
Time How long should we sustain these activities for?	Between 15 and 60 min is an optimal duration, with approximately 20 min being sufficient to maintain fitness. Less fit individuals would need to progress gradually to this duration. They may be better advised to follow the physical activity guidelines suggested in Part Two to build to this duration.
Type What types of activity are most effective?	Rhythmical, continuous activities that use the larger muscles and are aerobic (require oxygen) in nature. For example, walking, swimming, running, dancing, cycling and so on.

What are the long-term benefits of flexibility training?

Flexibility is essential for easing the performance of our everyday tasks. We need flexibility in our shoulder joints to reach our arms above our heads when we change a light bulb, or reach for an object on a high shelf. We need flexibility in our hip joints to lift our knees to climb stairs and take long strides when walking. If we are flexible we can move more efficiently.

Flexible joints and muscles also contribute to the maintenance of correct posture and joint alignment. Improved posture can potentially enhance our physical appearance and may reflect personal self-esteem. Standing tall and upright can provide a slimming effect to most body frames and can give the impression of the person being more confident. Flexibility also enables us to move with greater ease and greater poise.

If we lack flexibility our bodies become stiff and immobile. We will be less able to reach upwards or bend down to tie our shoelaces,

---

Summary of the long-term benefits of flexibility training

- Improved range of motion and mobility in the joints
- Improved length and range of movement achievable by the muscles
- Improved posture and skeletal alignment, which can assist with breathing and the functioning of internal organs
- Appearance of greater self-esteem and self-confidence
- Reduced muscular and physical tension
- Reduced risk of injury when moving into extended positions
- Enhanced performance of sporting and everyday activities

---

which can restrict the everyday movements we need to perform to maintain independence and self-sufficiency. Moving with an incorrect posture and joint alignment will potentially create muscle imbalance and increase joint and other mobility problems. Poor posture will also create a less aesthetically pleasing appearance. Flexibility is important for maintaining the quality and economy of our movements in everyday life.

How can we improve flexibility?

Regularly performing activities that require our muscles and joints to move through their full range of motion will maintain our flexibility. Most sedentary lifestyles do not provide this opportunity, therefore stretching and other exercise programmes to develop postural awareness such as stretch classes, yoga and Pilates need to be planned into our lives as part of a fitness regime.

Stretching activities are those that require the two ends of the muscle, the origin and insertion, to move further apart. This causes the muscle to lengthen, and will potentially increase the range of motion at the joint. The muscle must also be allowed to relax to achieve an effective stretch. Static stretch positions, where the muscle is held still at an extended length for a appropriate duration of time (from 10 to 30 seconds as a guideline), are generally advocated as safe for most people. This type of stretching will enable the tension initially felt in the muscle (the stretch reflex) to dissipate (desensitisation), which allows the muscle to relax and move more safely to an extended range of movement. Stretching in this way has the potential to improve our range of movement (flexibility). However, if we move too quickly or too far into the stretch (overstretch), then relaxation (desensitisation) of the muscle may not occur. It is therefore essential that we listen carefully to the body, and move only to the point of a mild tension.

Ballistic stretching movements, which require the body to move quickly into an extended range of motion, are more controversial for some individuals. This type of stretching can prevent desensitisation occurring and therefore potentially create muscle tearing and damage to the ligaments and other tissues surrounding the joint. They might also reduce the stability of the joints and create hypermobility (laxity or looseness of the ligaments around the joints), thereby causing irreparable damage to the muscles and joints, which might ultimately reduce the range of motion and decrease flexibility. While some sporting activities still include ballistic stretching as part of their training, static stretches are more appropriate for the general population.

Range-of-motion and dynamic stretches that involve lengthening the muscle at a more controlled speed through the full range of movement can be used, although it could be argued that they also do not allow sufficient time for the stretch reflex to desensitise. This would to some extent be dependent on the flexibility of the individual and the speed at which the movement is performed. Indeed, care must be taken not to move too quickly or too far into the stretch. If this occurs the stretch may become ballistic in nature and has the potential to cause injury. Ultimately, range of motion stretches are recommended only for persons with greater flexibility and higher levels of body awareness, otherwise the stretch will not be safe or effective. The recommended training requirements for improving flexibility are outlined in table 3.2.

Table 3.2 The recommended training requirements for improving flexibility	
Frequency How often should we perform these activities?	Before and after every training session are recommendations. Ideally, perform them every day to improve flexibility. The body *must* be warm prior to stretching to prevent muscle tearing and to enhance the range of motion achieved.
Intensity How hard should we be working?	Positions should allow the muscle to lengthen and relax and effect a slightly greater range of motion than is normally achievable.
Time How long should we sustain these activities for?	Stretch positions can be held from approximately 10–30 seconds. For greater improvements in flexibility longer durations are necessary.
Type What types of activity are most effective?	Positions that allow the targeted muscle to lengthen and relax, and the opposing muscle also to relax (passive static stretches) are most effective.

What is muscular strength and endurance?

Muscular strength is the ability of our muscles to exert a near maximal force to lift a resistance. Muscular endurance requires a less maximal force to be exerted, but for the muscle contraction to be maintained for a longer period.

What are the long-term benefits of muscular strength and endurance training?

We need a combination of muscular strength and endurance to carry out daily tasks that require us to lift, carry, pull, or push a resistance. Examples of these activities may include carrying shopping or children, digging the garden, moving furniture, climbing stairs and lifting ourselves out of a chair or bath.

This type of training will also improve muscle tone, which can make our body look firmer and more shapely and enhance physical appearance. If we perceive our body as being more toned and in shape this can enhance our physical self-esteem, which can improve our psychological well-being and self-confidence.

Improving muscular strength and endurance will maintain the health of our bones and joints. The muscles have to contract and pull against the bones to create movement, which can increase the calcium deposited and stored by the bone and prevent brittle bone disease (osteoporosis). The strength of the tendons, which attach muscle to bone, and of the ligaments, which attach bone to bone and keep the joints stable, will also improve. These benefits can enhance the physical quality of our life.

Balanced muscular strength will also help to maintain the correct skeletal alignment. Our muscles work in pairs – as one contracts and

works, the opposing muscle relaxes. If one of the pair is contracted or worked too frequently and becomes too strong and the other is not worked sufficiently or is allowed to become weaker, then our joints will be pulled out of the correct alignment. This can potentially cause injury, or create postural defects such as rounded shoulders or excessive curvatures of the spine, as illustrated in figure 3.1 overleaf. An imbalance of the strength between the abdominal and opposing muscles of the back (the erector spinae) can cause an exaggerated curve or hollowing of the lumbar vertebrae (lordosis). An imbalance of strength between the muscles of the chest (the pectorals) and the muscles between the shoulder blades (the rhomboids and trapezius) can cause rounded shoulders and a humping of the thoracic spine (kyphosis). An imbalance in strength between the muscles on each side of the back can cause a sideways curvature of the thoracic spine (scoliosis). All our muscles should therefore be kept sufficiently strong to maintain a correct

Summary of the long-term benefits of muscular strength and endurance training

- Increased bone density (more calcium deposited and stored by the bones)
- Reduced risk of osteoporosis (brittle bone disease)
- Improved posture and joint alignment
- Improved efficiency and performance of daily tasks, maintaining independence
- Improved body shape and tone
- Improved physical self-image
- Improved self-confidence
- Stronger muscles, ligaments and tendons, which are more supportive of movement
- Improved performance of sporting and recreational activities

Figure 3.1 Curvatures of the spine

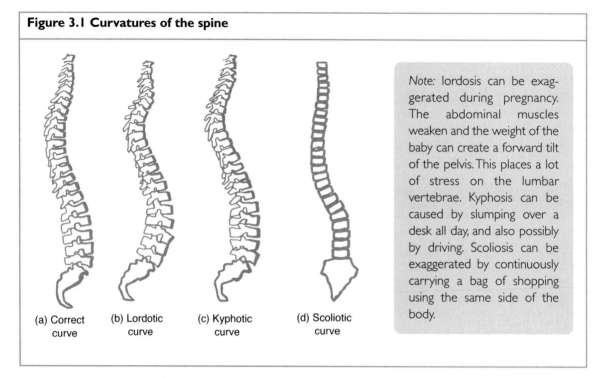

(a) Correct curve   (b) Lordotic curve   (c) Kyphotic curve   (d) Scoliotic curve

Note: lordosis can be exaggerated during pregnancy. The abdominal muscles weaken and the weight of the baby can create a forward tilt of the pelvis. This places a lot of stress on the lumbar vertebrae. Kyphosis can be caused by slumping over a desk all day, and also possibly by driving. Scoliosis can be exaggerated by continuously carrying a bag of shopping using the same side of the body.

posture. However, our lifestyle may demand that we specifically target certain muscles more than others to compensate for the imbalances caused by our work and daily activities. For the majority of persons with a sedentary lifestyle, it is well worth while strengthening the abdominal muscles, the muscles in between the shoulder blades (trapezius and rhomboids), and possibly the muscles of the back (erector spinae).

How do we improve our strength and endurance?

Strength training is traditionally achieved by performing exercises that require us to lift heavy and near-maximal resistances for a short period of time (high resistance and low repetitions). Endurance exercises require a lighter resistance to be lifted but for an extended period of time (lower resistance and higher repetitions). The type of activities that promote strength and endurance gains are those that require a more isolated focus on the specific muscles. These include:

- lifting weights (free weights or fixed resistance training);
- callisthenic exercises that require us to lift our body weight (e.g. press-ups, sit-ups);
- working with exercise bands and stability balls;
- exercising against the resistance of water.

These activities need to be performed approximately 2–3 times a week and the resistance lifted should promote a fatigued feeling in the muscle from anywhere between 7 and 25 repetitions approximately. Achieving muscle fatigue at lower repetitions will improve muscular strength predominantly. Achieving muscle fatigue at higher repetitions will improve muscular endurance predominantly.

The recommended training requirements for improving our muscular strength and muscular endurance are outlined in table 3.3.

Summary of the benefits of physical fitness

Developing our physical fitness will make a massive contribution to improving our overall health and total fitness. At a mental and emotional level, when we are exercising, our attention is distracted from daily hassles and worries; we literally take our minds off the problems and give them the rest they need by providing a more positive focus. The release of endorphins into the circulatory system can make us feel good and lift our spirits for much longer than the duration of the actual exercise session, which helps us manage other tasks more effectively.

At the physical, nutritional and medical levels, the exertion necessary to perform exercise provides an excellent release for the build-up of physical pressure and tension. It can trigger the processes needed to make use of the sugars that are released in our bodies when we become stressed and experience the fight or flight response, and will keep our heart and circulatory systems healthier, thus decreasing the risk of coronary heart disease and other diseases associated with stress and inactivity, such as diabetes, obesity, irritable bowel syndrome, high blood pressure, some cancers

Table 3.3	The recommended training requirements for improving muscular strength and muscular endurance
Frequency How often should we perform these activities?	Working the same muscle groups, 2–3 days per week.
Intensity How hard should we be working?	To improve strength, work with a greater resistance and lower repetitions (about 5–7). To improve endurance, work with a slightly lower resistance and slightly higher repetitions (about 12–25). Working with a resistance that allows a performance of 7–12 reps will provide some improvement in both strength and endurance.
Time How long should we sustain these activities for?	As a guideline, 20–40 min (excluding warm-up and warm-down) should be sufficent to achieve a whole body approach and train all the major muscle groups. This will depend on fitness and specific training goals.
Type What types of activity are most effective?	Lifting weights; working with body resistance; using other resistance equipment, such as bands or exercising in water.

and so on. Physical fitness will also keep our bones and joints healthy and prevent the onset of osteoporosis and other mobility conditions. It will keep our muscles strong and toned, which provides greater support to our skeleton and promotes physical independence. We will burn calories as we exercise and may also become more aware of our diet and sensitive to the types of food we are eating to provide fuel for the body, which can assist with our weight management and enhance our body image and physical self-esteem.

At a social level, if we feel secure about how we look we look our confidence increases, which can help to develop our social skills. Exercising with others provides opportunities to meet new people and develop our social skills and confidence. It can also create more opportunities to make friends, which adds to our life experience.

Each and every one of these benefits contributes, enables and creates potential for us to live a fuller life!

WORKING WITH THE WHOLE PERSON TO MANAGE STRESS

PART **TWO**

This section explores a range of potential resources we can access to assist with managing stress at a physical, behavioural, mental and emotional level. Each strategy may focus on one dimension but will tend to influence other aspects of the self. For example: using a relaxation technique may primarily release body tension, but will also ease mental tension and may soothe the emotions and thus influence our behaviour. The various strategies suggested in this section are intended to help build the resources we need to exercise away stress.

The model of total fitness is provided to highlight how a whole-person approach can manage stress more effectively. This model provides a goal to work towards. Personal trainers tend to focus and work on the physical aspect, while other professionals work on different aspects. Doctors will focus on the medical side, psychotherapists may work on various areas depending on the orientation of the psychological theories they follow, while a nutritionist will work on diet and eating regimes. Each professional has specific skills and experiences that they bring to manage each of the sections. Personal trainers should not consider themselves to be experts in all these areas, and should seek the support of other professionals to meet the needs of the client. Alternatively, they can take further training in each specific area to develop their knowledge and professional expertise. However, to become an expert in all the aspects of the model would be a lifelong journey of study. A more realistic way of working would be to establish connections with other organisations that provide a specific area of expertise (a multidisciplinary team) and share skills and knowledge to improve health and well-being, as all areas are interconnected. Table A provides an outline of the potential resources we can access in each component part.

Table A	A model of total fitness and potential resources we can access to manage stress

Physical fitness resources:
- Physical fitness (muscular strength, muscular endurance, flexibility, cardiovascular, motor skills)
- Posture
- Breathing
- Rest and sleep (do we enjoy undisturbed sleep?)

Factors affecting our physical fitness resources will include: physical differences; body type; body composition; gender; age and so on. (readers are directed towards other texts in the *Complete Guide* series for further information regarding specific physical fitness training programmes and factors affecting fitness)

Medical fitness resources:
- Being free from illness and injury
- Having access to appropriate healthcare

Nutritional fitness resources
Eating a healthy, balanced diet without an excess of caffeine, alcohol, salt, sugar, fat, fast food and so on

Mental fitness resources:
- Mental attitude ('I can handle' versus 'I cannot handle', 'I am good enough' versus 'I am not good enough', 'I will' versus 'I will not', 'I'm okay' versus 'I am not okay')
- Self-esteem (our thoughts and how they affect how we view our selves, others and life)
- Study skills (our intellect)
- Self-discipline and time management (our ability to prioritise and manage time effectively)

Emotional fitness resources:
Emotional awareness and intelligence (the feelings we allow ourselves to experience:
- Excitement–fear
- Calm–anger
- Joy–sadness
- Pleasure–pain
- Power–powerless

Emotional management and assertiveness (how we manage our emotional experience)

Spiritual fitness resources:
Having one's own beliefs, values and morals to help one through situations; these can include:
- Religious beliefs (Christian, Buddhist, Hindu, Moslem beliefs, etc.)
- Personal beliefs (our own values, morals, ethics, sense of self etc.)
- New age beliefs (paganism, universe etc.)

Social resources:
- Friends for socialisation and relaxation
- Relationship partners, family relationships and support
- Group memberships, training partners, study partners
- Other support groups (i.e. clubs for dieting, stopping smoking etc.)
- Financial resources and access to financial service management

STRATEGIES FOR MANAGING THE MENTAL AND EMOTIONAL SIGNS AND SYMPTOMS OF STRESS

4

In order to manage the mental and emotional signs and symptoms of stress, we need to be aware of what signs and symptoms we have developed that may be linked to stress. Table 4.1 provides a checklist for identifying some of these.

Table 4.1	Mental and emotional signs and symptoms checklist			
Mental		*Emotional cont.*	
Irrational thoughts		Fear	
Mental fatigue		Panic	
Poor decision-making		Irritability	
Low self-esteem		Boredom	
Low self-worth		Loneliness	
Inability to listen		Jealousy	
Procrastination (putting things off that need doing)		Resentment	
		Helplessness	
Excessive self-criticism		Powerlessness	
Egocentricity (focusing only on self)		Insecurity	
Accident proneness		Frustration	
Making more mistakes		Lethargy	
		Lack of focus	
Emotional		Tearfulness	
Sadness		Anxiety	
Anger		Loss of hope	
Depression			

What techniques are available to manage the mental and emotional signs and symptoms of stress?

There are many ways to combat the signs and symptoms of stress on a mental and emotional level; these, including:

- Building self-esteem and self-worth
- Positive self-talk and thinking strategies
- Meditation
- Being grateful
- Assertiveness
- Managing time
- Goal-setting
- Balancing life
- Building supportive social relationships
- Smiling and laughter
- Counselling and psychotherapy
- Worry time, hassle lists and possibility lists
- Self-help books
- Letting go of control
- Saying yes
- Managing fear and comfort zones
- Creative work
- Creature comforts.

Building self-esteem and self-worth

What is self-esteem?

Self-esteem is a state of mind; it is how you relate to and think about yourself. It is the value and worth that you place upon yourself.

If you have a high level of self-esteem, you will value your whole self (mind, emotions, body) and will make your decisions independently and assertively, trusting in yourself to be your own best friend. You will tend towards being optimistic, positive, self-reliant, well-nurtured, energetic and sensing your purpose in life.

If you have low self-esteem, you will place less value on your whole self. This can manifest in many ways: you may be judgemental and critical of yourself and others; you might not take care of your body or appearance; you might devalue your emotions, mistrust your own decisions, or seek relationships with others who will make your decisions for you.

> 'Self-esteem is the reputation we acquire with ourselves.'
>
> Nathaniel Branden

Self-esteem has a direct relationship to stress. People with a lower self-esteem will be more susceptible to destructive stress because of how they view the world and themselves. People with higher levels of self-esteem will be more 'hardy' and stress-proof in their nature.

Kobasa (1985) grouped together a number of factors that contribute to a person managing stress more effectively, giving them a more stress-proof or, as he suggested, a 'hardy' personality. Personal self-esteem and self-confidence were key factors, as was the willingness to be able to ask for help from appropriate life resource and support systems when needed. Other factors included commitment, challenge and control.

Commitment: Involving yourself fully and wholeheartedly in whatever task, activity or social event you are taking part in. Giving yourself 100 per cent to the task at hand.

For example: when you are walking or taking exercise, noticing how the muscles of your body are contracting, being fully aware; noticing if your mind starts to wander (i.e. thoughts turn to the rest of the day ahead or how you don't like this particular exercise etc.); being aware of

High self-esteem cycle

Your mind develops the belief that you are OK.
This makes you feel good about yourself and your confidence rises.
Your body responds by feeling relaxed, warm and energetic.
You feel attractive and content and this progressively leads to beliefs that the world is a safe place and your needs will be met.
This spirals to further positive beliefs that people are OK and trustworthy and the energy levels in your body rise again.
Your mind becomes lively and full of creative ideas and you take positive steps to get your needs met, which leads to further contentment, and you judge yourself as successful. The spiral continues.

Low self-esteem cycle

Your mind develops a belief that you are not OK.
This makes you feel bad about yourself and your confidence drops.
Your body responds by hunching over, tensing up, making itself smaller and less visible.
You feel unattractive and miserable and this progressively leads to beliefs that the world is not a nice place and your needs won't be met.
This spirals to further negative beliefs that other people are OK, it is just you that is not, and you wonder whether you are not a nice person.
You let other people take advantage of you and make your decisions, then become resentful and judge yourself as a horrible person for thinking such thoughts.
Your energy levels drop and your mind is full of negative and stressful thoughts.
You see yourself as unsuccessful and become more depressed.
The cycle keeps repeating until you commit to breaking it.

thoughts and letting yourself be fully present and focused on the current activity.

Challenge: Seeing life changes as naturally occurring phenomena that need to be responded to and viewing change as a positive event.

For example: life changes are guaranteed! We all move through different life events such as potty training, starting school, making friends etc. These changes continue throughout life. The key is how we respond to changes. Each change brings a new experience to learn from.

Control: Believing that, whatever life brings, you have the power to influence events (an internal locus of control) by taking responsibility and making choices. The alternative to this is to view all life situations as out of your control (an external locus of control) and that you are a victim of fate with little power to manage what happens to you.

For example: losing a job or relationship. We can make the choice to hold on to the disappointment and other feelings we have in relation to this loss and the impact it has on our sense of self. Alternatively, we can release and work through these feelings and allow space for energy to motivate us to move forward and make other changes in ourselves and our lives.

What factors determine a person's level of self-esteem?

Babies enter the world as perfect little beings with equal potential for developing a higher level of self-esteem. When children start school, they will have already experienced some of the effects of living in the world (these are listed in Chapter 1) and there are noticeable differences in the confidence of young children when they arrive for their first day at school. The socialisation process continues and we receive a combination of positive and negative strokes to ourselves from other significant sources such as parents, friends, teachers, partners, the media, employers – and this in turn will both increase and decrease our confidence.

If we receive too many negative strokes or we learn to focus on the negative strokes we will develop a lower self-esteem. If we receive more positive strokes or we learn to focus on the positive strokes then our self-esteem will be higher. The positive aspect of this is that we cannot change the socialisation process we have experienced, but we can change how we respond to these experiences. Self-esteem can be relearned to serve us more positively and healthily.

Indeed, like all aspects of the self, self-esteem is not a permanent and steady state; it needs to be worked continuously by performing life- and personal growth-enhancing activities. Some of these activities are listed in Table A on page 27.

Why do we need a high level of self-esteem?

This is almost a ridiculous question because a high level of self-esteem is essential to our overall health. The way we think about ourselves links closely with our emotional and physical well-being. It has already been discussed how our 'stressful' thinking can affect our bodies. If we think uncomfortable thoughts about ourselves, this will only compound the problems. A high self-esteem will impact and improve:

- Health and well-being
- Emotional confidence
- Stress levels
- Personal motivation
- Personal success
- Creativity
- Depression
- Relationships

- Interest and purpose in life
- Personal happiness.

How do we develop a higher level of self-esteem?

There are numerous ways in which we can build our self-esteem and self-worth. The key to success is making a start and to keep working on ourselves. Table 4.2 overleaf provides some strategies for developing self-esteem.

A final point on self esteem is that many people attach their personal self-esteem to other external things. For example:

Appearance: Some people attach self-esteem to personal attractiveness and how others see them.

Education: Some people attach self-esteem to what qualifications and knowledge they have.

Materialistic success: Some people attach self-esteem to the car they drive and the home they live in.

Work: Some people attach self-esteem to the job they do, the organisation they work for or what they do for others.

Social circle: Some people attach self-esteem to the people they know or different groups they belong to.

Partner: Some people attach self-esteem to their partner.

Performance: Some people attach self-esteem to how well they perform, and have to put on a personal show to prove they are OK.

These things are important aspects that may contribute to our self esteem. The problem arises when we attach too much personal esteem to these things and become dependent on them for a sense of well-being. If they fall away, what then?

Self-esteem is knowing internally that we are valuable and worthwhile no matter what. It is about accepting ourselves totally and embracing who we are.

Table 4.2	Strategies for developing self-esteem

Control your mind
- Use positive self-talk and positive affirmations
- Write positive affirmations about your life and the things you have to be grateful for
- Notice all the positive things that happen in your life. In her book *Feel the Fear and Do It Anyway* Susan Jeffers suggests writing 50 positive things each day. It is an achievable and immensely valuable activity!
- Remember that if we have thousands of thoughts each day, it is better to make them positive ones
- You have the power to manage your mind and make it your best friend

Develop positive habits
- Meditation
- Breathing
- Activity
- Exercise
- Eating
- Sleep

Manage your time between all life priorities and give 100 per cent of yourself to each at specific times:
- Self
- Friends
- Family
- Social life
- Partner
- Work
- Home
- Study

Keep promises made to yourself
- Set realistic goals that you can achieve
- Reward yourself as you achieve your goals
- Praise yourself every step of the way

Be nice to others
- Treat people how you would like them to treat you
- Smile
- Send positive thoughts to others
- Give without the expectation of receiving
- Notice the nice things others do for you
- Say thank you
- Show appreciation and value for others

Change your vision
- See stress as a challenge, not as a problem

Table 4.2	Strategies for developing self-esteem cont.

Accept responsibility
- Own your feelings
- Use 'I' statements when you speak and express your feelings
- Avoid blaming others

Visualise
- Picture yourself as you would like to be
- Picture your life how you want it to be

Because I am the only person I will have a relationship with all my life, I choose:
To love myself the way I am now
To always acknowledge that I am enough just the way I am
To love, honor and cherish myself
To be my own best friend
To be the person I would like to spend the rest of my life with
To always take care of myself so that I can take care of others
To always grow, develop and share my love and life.

Author unknown.
(From: J. Roger and P. McWilliams (1990) – You Can't Afford the Luxury of a Negative Thought)

Mind awareness activity

Stop what you are doing and become aware of the thoughts entering your mind. If you think to yourself, 'I'm not thinking anything', then recognise this is a thought! So to think you are thinking nothing would be incorrect.

Just stay aware of all the thoughts that go through your mind and notice how well you speak to yourself. Do this regularly and you will start becoming aware of how you think.

Some thoughts may be positive: I really worked well today; I had an enjoyable day. Some thoughts may be negative: I am so stupid; I really don't like myself. Some thoughts may just be neutral thoughts: What shall I have for dinner?

Self-esteem boost

Repeat this phrase to yourself 20 times:
'I value and believe in myself.'

Positive self-talk and thinking strategies

A key step towards developing self-esteem and taking care of our mental and emotional well-being is to become aware of the way we speak to ourselves and the messages we send ourselves internally. Most people's response to the notion of having little voices that chatter in our heads would be to consider this crazy. However, the voices are there and they are fairly natural. Try the mind awareness activity below.

Another technique is just being aware of the words you use to describe yourself throughout the day. When you drop something: 'I'm so clumsy'; when you look in the mirror: 'I'm so fat and ugly'; when you make a mistake: 'I'm so stupid and such a fool'. Start listening to what you say to yourself and the message this sends to your mind and heart.

Being aware of how your mind works is a key to making yourself your own best friend. If you constantly look at things negatively or the glass seems half empty rather than half full then it would be wise if you took particular care of this aspect of your well-being.

> *'Every good thought you think is contributing its share to the ultimate result of your life.'*
>
> *Grenville Kleiser*

Our thoughts pass through our minds so quickly, it is no wonder that most of our self-talk is beyond our awareness. Those people who are aware of their thinking some of the time are more than halfway towards improving their situation. The way we think really makes a difference, as it acts like a self-fulfilling prophecy: the more we see something as bad or awful, the worse it gets! Whereas if we can stop our thought processes before we get carried away and create a whole negative story, then we may be able to see more positives in the situation. The art of positive thinking is, as Louise Hay suggests, about faking it till you make it! That is, think positive thoughts, even if you don't believe them at first. If you keep putting positive thoughts in, then positive comes out. If you choose to put negative thoughts in, then all you will see is negative.

Look in the box below and make a note of what you see.

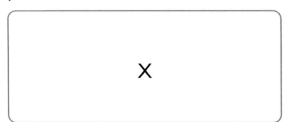

Did you see the whole box of empty space? Or did you see the X in the middle? Both are there, it is our focus that counts. It could be that only a small part of your life is negative, represented by the X, and that most of your life is positive like the empty space surrounding the X. The key is where we allow our mind to focus! Becoming aware of your mind and of the way you think is the first step to changing your focus. Furthermore, developing a positive mental attitude towards life events has an impact on our emotions and how we feel. If we think positive thoughts, we tend to feel better. If we think negative thoughts, it is hardly surprising that our life seems 'doom and gloom'. A further factor is that how we feel can impact our ability to take action. If we think negatively and feel bad, we will perceive powerlessness and this will reduce our energy levels and our action potential. Whereas if we think positively, we will feel better, and this will raise our energy levels, giving us more potential to take action.

Ask any person who has experienced an episode of depression how that felt. It would have taken a tremendous mental effort from them to make the first step to lift themselves out of that low mood and take action to improve their situation. Often people require external psychological support to provide motivation and encouragement – personal training for the mind! However, making the first step is the key to recovery and to moving forward to make positive changes.

Instant stress relief

Repeat this phrase 20 times:

'I am a positive and powerful human being!'

Table 4.3	Negative and positive viewpoints
Negative	**Positive**
I only have one week left of my holiday and then I have to go back to work.	I am only halfway through my holiday, I still have a whole week left.
I'm so stupid for letting that person be so rude to me.	I would like to be treated more respectfully by that person so I will assert myself next time I speak with them. (NB: this doesn't mean the person will respond positively to your assertions. The key is that you can then decide whether she or he is the type of person you want to spend time with.)
I hate working weekends.	The positive thing about working weekends is that I can go shopping in the week when it is much quieter.
I really don't like exercising.	I like exercising, I feel so much better once I've finished my workout.

Meditation

Short meditation script

- Sit comfortably with an open posture.
- Close your eyes.
- Focus on breathing deeply and slowly for a count of 10.
- Become aware of the activity of your mind and the speed of your thoughts.
- Let the thoughts pass through your mind – let them go.
- Focus on stillness.
- Focus on allowing the mind to slow down.
- Focus on letting the mind become quiet and silent.
- If you are tempted to hold on to any particular thought, be aware of that thought.
- Acknowledge that you have heard that thought, smile and let it go, release the thought just for now.
- Bring your attention back to focusing on the stillness, allowing the mind to slow down, letting the mind rest and become quiet and silent.
- Allow your mind to be clear and peaceful.

Instant stress relief

If your mind feels harried, take 5 minutes to sit quietly and complete the short mind meditation script listed above. This short meditation can be used to start your day and end your day.

If you find yourself particularly overwhelmed by thoughts, write them down on paper (you may prefer to draw a picture or a doodle – see the section on creative work on pages 52–6). Avoid judging the thoughts, just let them come out on paper.

Once you have written them down, take a look at all the things that fill your mind. Notice how many of these thoughts are positive and how many are negative. You can change that balance. Awareness is the key to making changes!

Being grateful and showing appreciation

Another strategy for building self-esteem and reducing stress levels is to start noticing all the things in life you take for granted because they are always there. There is a saying, 'You don't know what you've got until its gone'. This is so true, and relates to so many areas of life. It is often much easier to focus negatively on all the things we don't have and want that we forget to notice what we have and appreciate and value those things. Health is one example! So many people ignore their health until illness pervades and they have to take notice.

At a more simple level, there is so much that we take for granted: running fresh water, central heating, electricity, gas, having a home, having a car, having friends, being able to walk and talk, being able to read and write, having trees and flowers (these don't exist in a desert), having a washing machine and freezer (these things make our lives so much easier), having food to eat.

> 'The mind is its own place, and in itself can make a heaven of hell, and a hell of heaven.'
>
> Milton

Write a grateful list

List 10 things you are grateful for having in your life. Progress this number gradually and see how much you can increase your focus on to what you have to be grateful for.

You can make this a daily activity. It is amazingly powerful and levelling.

NB: One client of mine has written a diary for a number of years. Each day she writes down one thing that has touched each of her senses. She reports that it is really great to look back and review the things she has found value in on the days when she feels stressed.

Assertiveness

Another strategy to assist with managing stress and improving self-esteem is learning to be assertive. The first step towards developing assertiveness is to recognise your own rights and the rights of others. These are listed in the box below.

A second step in improving your assertiveness is to recognise when you and others may be behaving non-assertively. There are three main ways of behaving non-assertively, which are listed in table 4.4. We can all behave unassertively at times, but the key is to recognise how often and how this affects us, then we can make changes.

Further information on the behaviours listed in table 4.5 can be found in numerous other texts, some of which are listed as further reading.

Assertiveness rights

Each individual (this includes both yourself and others) has the right to:

Ask for what they want (appreciating that the other person has the right to say NO).

Say no.

Have and express their opinions, feelings and thoughts appropriately.

Make their own decisions and manage the consequences.

Change their mind.

Private time.

Be successful.

Not to know about something.

Choose whether to get involved with the problems of another.

Make mistakes.

Say: 'I don't understand.'

Be treated with respect.

Act assertively or choose not to do so.

NB: A fuller list of assertive rights can be found in Bayne et al., *Counsellors Handbook* (1998:7).

Table 4.4	Non-assertive behaviours		
	Manipulative	*Aggressive*	*Passive*
Attitude	I'm OK, you're not OK but I'll let you think you're OK	I'm OK You're not OK	I'm not OK You're OK
General	Manipulative Deceitful Sneaky Charming	Domineering Judgemental Punitive Hostile Insensitive Controlling	Meek Submissive Compliant Helpless Pessimistic
Personal power	Lets others think they have power by being sneaky	Controls others	Gives in to others
Emotions	Fearful Feigning other emotions to cover up the fear	Resentful Angry Raging Excitable Lonely	Fearful Anxious Depressed Bitter Guilty
Language	If you Why don't you	You should You had better I told you so You make me feel Stupid, bad	I guess I wonder You know It's only me Sorry to bother you
Body language	Upright posture Direct eye contact Fake smile	Hands on hips Head forward Staring Loud voice Clenched fists Finger-pointing	Stooped posture Looking down Whining voice Soft-spoken
Lifestyle	Most of energy used covering up deceit and game-playing	Fast Competitive	Safe Uneventful Low-risk
Gains	Plays games to get what is wanted	Seeks authority and control	Looks for attention or sympathy
Costs	Loss of respect and trust	Loss of friendship and love	Loss of self-respect and freedom

Table 4.5	Assertive behaviour
	Assertive
Attitude	I'm OK, you're OK
General	Optimistic, thoughtful, positive, sensitive, compromising, self-protective
Personal power	Shares power and can be vulnerable
Emotions	Full range of emotions experienced: joy, sadness, anger, fear
Language	I want, I feel, I don't like, I love, let's discuss, no, yes
Body language	Upright posture, direct eye contact, clear voice, expressive
Lifestyle	Varied, dynamic, purposeful, ethical
Gains	Self-respect and integrity
Costs	Unrealistic expectation to be perfectly assertive all the time

Once you have explored ways in which you are behaving non-assertively, you can take steps towards developing your assertiveness. Table 4.5 describes assertive behaviour.

How to be more assertive

Decide want you want: make sure you know what you want and be persistent in reinforcing this.

State what you want clearly and specifically: make sure your voice tone and body language match the words you use. It is no use stating what you want assertively if your body language is hunched and apologetic. Know that you have the right to ask for what you want and ask assertively.

Use I statements: 'I' statements are empowering. 'You' statements are blaming. (See Table 4.6.)

Listen to the other person: let the other person respond and listen with the intention of reading between the lines. Clarify back to the person what you hear them say and what you notice.

Table 4.6	'I' and 'you' statements
I feel angry . . .	You are making me feel angry . . .
I would like . . .	You should . . .
I think . . .	You think . . .

Stay focused: do not allow others to sidetrack or confuse you.

Aim for a win–win situation: there may be times when you do not get what you want. Sometimes a compromise is workable and maybe there is the opportunity to discuss this. If you find yourself permanently in a situation where you feel your rights are dismissed or ignored, it may be worth exploring other avenues and alternative ways of getting your needs met. However, it is advisable not to use this as a method of manipulation.

Manage your feelings: recognise your feelings in a situation and be comfortable with and take care of these. You can choose to express your feelings in an empowering way by owning them and embracing them, for example 'I feel hurt when I think you do not hear me', or you can choose not to express your feelings at that time and talk them through with a friend or other support person later. Bear in mind that people will not always respond positively, despite your efforts. The key is to manage and take care of your own well-being and be respectful of your rights and the rights of the other person.

Practise: keep practising and know that sometimes you may get it wrong. Be patient and learn from these experiences. Sometimes it can be useful to rehearse a dialogue with a friend to practise what you want to say in a specific situation.

For example: Case study 2 (see Part Four) frequently gets asked to stay late at work on a Friday evening when she has another appointment. She wants to be able to say NO to her boss. She worries about saying NO and this leads her into feeling fearful and taken for granted.

Practising the dialogue in Table 4.7 and experiencing the feelings that go along with the dialogue can help with managing the situation. In the practice dialogue, the client reinforces that she has an appointment and is valuing a commitment to herself and prioritising her needs equally. She is also acknowledging the importance of the task to the other person and has offered a couple of alternatives that she can work with, which are acceptable to her. Her boss may or may not appreciate her assertiveness. The key is that she has expressed herself assertively and given herself rights and respect in the situation.

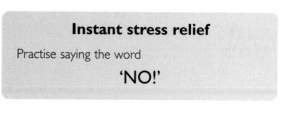

Instant stress relief

Practise saying the word

'NO!'

Managing time

Time is precious and it is essential that we balance our time between all life demands equally and make enough time to take care of

Table 4.7	Example of how to say 'no'
Friend (acting as boss):	Can you finish this before you go?
Client:	No, I can't today. I have an appointment at 5.30.
Friend:	It will only take five minutes.
Client:	I have an appointment at 5.30 today. It will take longer than five minutes. I appreciate it is important to you. I have to get to my appointment. I can complete it on Monday.
Friend:	I need it done now.
Client:	I have an appointment at 5.30. I can do it first thing Monday morning. If in future you give it to me earlier, I can complete it before I go to my appointment.

ourselves and spend time doing things we love with people we love in the process. This will assist with managing stress.

In order to manage time effectively we need to make sure that we are able to:

- Identify our priorities and share our time equally among these;
- Recognise less important, time-wasting activities;
- Not take on more than we can handle (say NO);
- Delegate tasks or ask for help and support if needed;
- Make time for ourselves, and for activities we enjoy that will help to manage stress.

Identifying priorities

The first step is to become aware of how we use our time. Using a 24-hour recall of what we did the previous day can be one way of recognising this. This can be used to raise awareness of how we spend our time at work and our leisure time.

Again, it can be useful to sit down with a friend, partner or even a manager at work to look at different strategies to help manage time more effectively. You may want to explore at what times of the day you feel most productive, or the ways in which you waste time; the things you do to manage time effectively, and what things you would like to change, if any.

Strategies for using time more effectively

Write a list: making a list of things that need to get done and ordering the priority of their importance is useful for managing time. Tackle the important things that you dislike doing first so that they get done and are not overlooked or carried over onto the following day's list (for listaholics!)

How do you use your time?

1. Write a list of all the things you did the previous day.
2. Make a note of how long they took to complete.
3. Make a note of whether these activities were:
   (a) Very important
   (b) Important
   (c) Not important
   (d) Time-wasting
   (e) Could have been delegated.

If there are too many a's on your list, you are probably overloaded and need to ask for some support or delegate some tasks. Alternatively, you may need to learn to say NO and not take on more than you can handle.

If there were lots of d's on your list, it may be worth reflecting on ways to minimise these and use your time more productively. (NB: a 10-minute relaxation is NOT a waste of time in your day, neither is taking time out to exercise or meet with a friend).

If there are a lot of e's on your list, reflect on why you keep these jobs for yourself and look at ways you could delegate and get help.

Tackle one task at a time: set an achievable time-frame (goal-setting) for getting things done and reward yourself at each stage.

Telephones: put your phone on silent and use an answer phone. Set a specific time of the day when you will deal with calls.

Interruptions from other people: whether at home or at work, establish rules that when your office door or your private room space is closed, you do not want to be interrupted. NB: At home your private space could be for completing a college assignment in your home office or taking time out to relax in the bath. Either way, you do not want to be interrupted and deserve to have some time out for yourself.

Perfectionism: striving to complete work perfectly can create additional stress and time wasting and may not enhance the quality of work. Establish a workable standard that you can achieve and time to reflect and review on work at a later date, with the help of others.

Emails: set a time each day when you will check and respond to emails.

Routine: establish a disciplined routine for things that you want to get done but can easily put off. This varies from one individual to another but can include things such as making time to exercise, paying bills, completing accounts and bookwork, cleaning the house and so on.

Pace yourself: know the times of the day when you feel more productive and the times when you feel more tired. Save the activities that you love doing for your tired time as these will lift your mood.

NO: learn how to say the NO word! Practise saying it in front of a mirror! Practise shouting it out (in private!). Practise saying NO without giving an excuse or reason as to why you are saying NO! If necessary, take an assertiveness training course to help you or read the assertiveness guidelines provided at the beginning of this chapter. Saying no is the key to making sure you do not take on more than you are able to handle. If in doubt, use the affirmation 'It is OK for me to say NO', and repeat this regularly.

Breaks: schedule regular breaks and time-out intervals during the day to relax and refuel. A high carbohydrate snack can help to keep the brain alert and maintain sugar level balance. A short relaxation exercise or some desk mobility exercises can clear the mind and release tension from the body, helping you to work more efficiently! If you miss your break or work through breaks, this can make you feel more pressured and mentally tired.

Advance meal planning: cooking meals and freezing them is a useful way of planning meals and saving time.

Paying other people: employing a cleaner or paying the kids extra pocket money can be a method of delegating household chores. Consider employing a typist to type up college assignments if you cannot type.

There are many other ways of saving time and using the time you have effectively. Sometimes all that is needed is the opportunity to take some time out to plan effectively, rather than rushing around and doing things in every spare minute. Make times when you can just sit and reflect and plan your time more carefully. Above all, make time to spend doing things that you enjoy that are just for you. The 'time out for you' activity listed below is a good way of getting started.

Activity: Time out for you

How much time do you get just for yourself to do what you want to do without interruption?

Make a note of what you could do if you had the following time frames free:

If I had a free 10 minutes I would . . .

If I had a free hour I would . . .

If I had a free half day I would . . .

If I had a whole day free I would . . .

Sit and chat with a friend or colleague to identify ways of making more time for yourselves.

Stress relief

Book an appointment in your diary for yourself and use it to do exactly what you would like to do, for example: go swimming, to hairdressers, to meditation class etc.

Make these self appointments more regular!

Goal-setting

Goal-setting can be a positive way of making changes and establishing appropriate time-frames for getting things done and reducing stress levels.

Using the SMART method can help to make goals workable:

Specific – decide what you want

Measurable – how will you know you are succeeding?

Achievable – is your goal possible?

Reward yourself – treat yourself as you achieve

Time-framed – set time limits for goals.

Specific: To relax for 10 minutes on 3 days per week.

Measurable: I can measure the above.

Achievable: I can identify blocks to my achieving 10 minutes on 3 days per week and adapt my goal accordingly.

Reward: How can I reward myself when I achieve my goal?

Time: When do I want to achieve this goal by?

Stress relief

Think about something you would like to do or achieve.

Make it a goal using the SMART format.

Balancing life

Another strategy for managing stress is to keep our lives full and interesting. It is important that we have a variety of things in our life to maintain stability and balance. Susan Jeffers suggests using a grid of life boxes (tables 4.8 and 4.9) to keep our lives full. If all these boxes are full, then if one falls away there is still a range of other things that add purpose to your life.

Allowing one single area to become emotionally consuming can lead to additional fear and stress. If all your focus is on one thing, for example work or children or relationships, and you make little time for the other areas in your life, then if that thing falls away, your life will

Table 4.8	Life boxes		
Study	Exercise	Friends	Work/career
Relaxation	Personal and spiritual growth	Family	Social
Nutrition	Contribution	Relationship	Home

Table 4.9	Use this chart to develop your own boxes		

feel empty indeed. For example, mothers or fathers may focus all their attention on their children, as depicted by the box below. When the children, grow and leave the nest there would be a big empty space to fill.

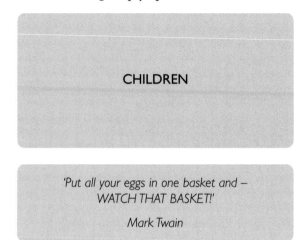

CHILDREN

'Put all your eggs in one basket and – WATCH THAT BASKET!'

Mark Twain

In addition to this, you would be lacking some of the other important support systems that help us make it through stressful times.

Another important aspect is to commit yourself 100 per cent to each area. For example, when with your partner, be totally with her or him and not worrying about other things or doing work. When you are exercising, focus totally on the workout and avoid thinking of all the other things you have to do. Be fully focused and committed to each area.

A final way of using the grid of life to reduce stress is to add a box marked 'contribution' and make yourself part of something much larger than yourself. A personal example of this is that I volunteer one afternoon each week to work as a psychotherapist with clients experiencing depression. I can be very introspective and focus very much on myself and on occasions be unaware of what is going on around me. Hearing my clients speak, noticing their discomfort and watching them make steps to move forward with their lives is one of the most

rewarding things I have ever experienced. It helps me to realise that I do make a difference and that everything I do is important.

Create a wish list

Often we can become stressed because we are dealing with the daily, run-of-the-mill activities and not exploring our dreams. There may be many unfulfilled dreams and desires inside our hearts. One way of exploring what these are is to make a wish list of all the things you would like and want to achieve. A wish list can be used to formulate goals for making things happen or it can be used as a vision of what you may like in your life. I write a wish list every year and at the end of the year I notice which of my wishes have come true and which ones are still on the list that I would still like to fulfil. When I write my wish list I let my imagination run wild and put everything I think I would like on the list. I am fairly relaxed about my list. I don't allow it to drive me excessively. There are always some things I would like to achieve and it tends to work out that I focus on these first, and usually get some of my wishes coming true. The wishes that haven't come true I review and I add them on to my next year's wish list. I don't give myself a hard time about the wishes that don't come true, I just notice them and explore any blocks I may have to making them come true. Sometimes I notice it is a fear or a belief inside myself that prevents that wish from materialising. This allows me the opportunity to work with those aspects in myself. I also value that some of my wishes may actually be reminders from my subconscious to work on that aspect of myself, they may not actually be about materialising the actual wish.

When I write my wish list I allow myself to be unspecific and unfocused. I can use the SMART goal-setting strategy if I want to focus on achieving a particular item. However, I have also found that just creating the wish and letting it go can also help me to get some of the things I would like. There have been a few occasions when I have written a wish, forgotten about it and months later it arrives. I believe this is my subconscious way of working towards the things that are really important to me.

Wish list

Buy a beach house in Brazil
Take a course in Jungian psycho-analysis
Make more time for myself to relax (hot baths with candles etc.)
Improve my eating patterns
Have more social events with friends
Do something different each day
Get some new writing projects
Pass my college assignments
Allow myself to be happy
Pay off my mortgage
Keep my car clean
Make time for others and not be too busy

'You see things and you say "Why?" But I dream things that never were and I say "Why not?"'

George Bernard Shaw

Building supportive relationships

A key factor in assisting with the management of stress is to have a good range of personal support systems, such as friends and family.

'One's friends are that part of the human race with which one can be human'

George Santayana

Many of the clients I work with in a counselling setting indicate they have low support systems in the form of friendships. This is frequently linked to low self-esteem, poor assertiveness and the belief that other people are too busy or have their own lives and may not want or need friends etc. The irony of these negative beliefs and attitudes is that they affect a number of people who I have worked with and that by reaching out to make friends the person(s) would find some of the support they need. They would also recognise that other people frequently experience the same inner dilemmas! It is easy to think and feel that you are the only one experiencing a problem, which compounds the feeling of aloneness. The benefit of reaching out and communicating with other people is that frequently we recognise that we are not alone and that many other people experience similar stresses and occurrences. It is a human need to feel connected and part of something. Connection can be found with family, friends, at work, at an exercise class, at an evening study course and so on.

'The meeting of two personalities is like the contact of two chemical substances: if there is any reaction, both are transformed.'

Carl Jung

Smiling and laughter

Smiling and laughter have a positive effect on how we feel about ourselves. If you feel miserable or stressed, try smiling for one minute; it reduces the negative tension around the face, relaxes the facial muscles and often brings about a more positive feeling. If you have forgotten how to smile, start adding smiles to your daily routine. Fake it till you make it!

Stress relief

Think of something you have always wanted to study or take part in and find a class in your local area. Ideas include:

Amateur dramatics
An art class
A photography class
A psychology class
A history class
Poetry appreciation
Pottery class
Sculpture class
Astrology group
An exercise class
A running club
A walking group
A cookery class
A language class

This will bring you into contact with other people who share a common interest and can help to provide other interests.

'Treat yourself to a facelift – smile.'

Richard Wilkins

Laughter is an incredible way of reducing stress. While a good belly laugh will initially elevate heart rate, blood pressure and muscle tension, these will drop significantly after the laughter ends, providing an instant feel-good. A great way of creating laughter is to have some of your favourite comedy videos in your home collection for the days when you feel low. Just put one on and let yourself laugh away the stress and increase your positive feelings. TV is usually filled with negative events going on in the world, it is OK to take a break from these and use your leisure time to focus on films that create pleasure.

I have found that when I speak through some of my problems and stresses with friends and they listen attentively, I frequently end up laughing at my own seriousness. I can lose my humour and perspective when I feel bogged down in stress. Talking and laughter can really help me gain perspective.

Instant stress relief

SMILE!
It reduces lots of tension around the face.
You feel better when you smile (a genuine, warm smile, not a grimace).
It can also make others feel better.
Smiling is a gift!

LAUGH!
Laughter is a great exercise for the deeper abdominal muscles.
When was the last time you laughed so much your belly ached?
Aim to laugh at least once a day – laughter is a great medicine, as Robert Holden (1999) suggests.

Self-help books and tapes

There are numerous self-help books and tapes available to manage stress, improve self-esteem and help with management of emotions. These books are written in a way that is aimed to inspire and motivate. However, some individuals will find some books useful while other books may be irritating to them. The best idea is to go into a bookshop and explore the different books on the shelves and notice what books attract you personally. Some of the self-help books that inspired the writing of this book in some way are listed as further recommended reading on pages 146–7.

Counselling and psychotherapy

Counselling and psychotherapy are excellent ways for getting to know your mind and emotions better and moving towards making better decisions for yourself. Counselling can be used to develop self-esteem and help with managing stressful situations. Many people may still hold the view that the use of these services is for persons with mental health distress. These services can be and are used for persons with distress of the mind. They can also be viewed and used as a method of personal training for the mind and achieving personal growth.

Friends and family may not always have the time or the skills to listen and hear problems and concerns effectively. They also have a personal involvement in a person's history, which can make them less objective. A therapist is professionally trained to listen actively and use different skills and techniques to reflect what they hear, see and sense. They also follow a code for ethical practice with the priority being the needs and wants of the client. There are many different types of therapy; some of these approaches may work better for different people. Some of the core approaches are described below.

Psychodynamic therapy

This type of therapy is generally long-term in nature. Sometimes clients visit from two to five times a week. It requires dedication and commitment from the clients and a reasonable level of self-awareness and ability to reflect. It is less appropriate for clients wishing to work on an immediate crisis.

Psychodynamic therapy has evolved from the earlier psychoanalytical work of Freud. The key themes explored in this work include:

- the unconscious
- personality structure (Id, Ego and Superego)

- psychosexual development (oral, anal, phallic, latency, genital)
- childhood experiences.
- defence mechanisms (denial, projection, rationalisation, introjection, regression etc.)
- transference and counter-transference
- dreams
- free association
- interpretation.

Other theories that have evolved from this school include: Carl Jung's analytical psychology; Melanie Klein and other object relations theorists; Erikkson's psychosocial stages of development; Kohut's theory of self-psychology, and many other theories.

Cognitive therapy

This approach works well with clients who want to work on a specific problem in a directive manner, for an established time-frame. It is appropriate for clients who lack assertiveness or need to build personal esteem and change thinking patterns. It would not be appropriate for clients wanting to explore deeper aspects of their psyche. Additionally, some people may find the approach too directive.

There are different schools of cognitive therapy. One of the most popular models is Rational Emotive Behavior therapy, which was pioneered by Albert Ellis in 1955. Ellis (see Feltham and Horton 2000) noticed that clients tended to cling to negative thinking patterns that reinforced disturbing experiences and were outdated in the present. He recognized how the language and internal dialogue used by clients would reinforce old anxieties and fears, therefore people were largely responsible for their own feelings and thus had the power within them to create changes. Ellis produced the ABC model of personality, which links how a person's beliefs in response to a situation can influence their feelings and behaviour.

For example:

Activating event (something happens): Jane's friend says she is busy on Tuesday evening and cannot go to see a movie.

Beliefs (rational or irrational): Jane decides this person is rejecting her and is not really a friend.

Consequences (emotional and behavioural): Jane feels depressed.

Ellis's therapy was directive and focused on working with the ABC model to work towards challenging beliefs: For example:

Activating event (something happens): Jane's friend says she is busy on Tuesday evening and cannot go to see a movie.

Beliefs (rational or irrational): Jane decides it would be nice if they could spend time together at some stage but that her friend has the right to do other things too.

Consequences (emotional and behavioural): Jane feels OK and makes a new plan with her friend at another time.

Ellis identified a number of irrational beliefs that an individual may hold. An adapted version of some of these includes:

- I should always be loved and approved of by everybody.
- I have to be good at everything to be worthwhile.
- All bad people should be punished, including myself.
- It is a disaster if things don't go my way.
- External events are the cause of my problems, I have no control.
- I have to have someone strong to look after me.

Ellis also noticed how his clients used the words 'should', 'must' and 'ought', which placed high demands on themselves. For example: 'relationships should be...' and 'all people should...' and 'I must do this...'.

Recognising one's own irrational beliefs

Work with a close friend or partner and take a look at the irrational beliefs listed opposite. See which ones you may have in the past subscribed to and explore their origins and impact on your experience.

You can also explore your general beliefs around specific area, such as:

Work
Relationships
Success and power
Sex
Love
Men and women
Money

If you write down all your beliefs about these areas, you can explore which ones are negative and which are positive and work towards making changes to the former.

Changing the shoulds and musts

If these words are replaced with the word COULD, it gives the person a choice and helps them take responsibility for their decisions.

Notice how often you use the words MUST and SHOULD. Experiment with using the word COULD and notice how that feels and if it changes how you experience things, and how it impacts your stress levels.

Humanistic therapy

This type of therapy offers respect, understanding and openness, and facilitates the client to find her or his own answers. It works effectively for persons experiencing loss, bereavement or relationship problems. It is the model most frequently used by other helping professions. It may not be helpful for people who prefer a directive approach and want more specific interventions.

There are a number of humanistic schools of thinking. A key model is the person-centred approach pioneered by Carl Rogers. Rogers (1967) believed that each person was the creator of her or his own destiny and had the resources within to deal with all the obstacles that living presents. He believed that within each person was an innate sense of being, the 'organismic self', which would never be obliterated and always had the potential to become. He proposed that with the right conditions (empathy, unconditional positive regard and congruency) and in the right environment people would move towards finding their organismic self and move towards autonomy and self-directedness.

The person-centred approach is based on the relationship between the client and therapist and is less directive in nature than cognitive therapy. Techniques used by these therapists include: active listening, paraphrasing, summarising, reflecting feelings and content and asking open questions. Some of these techniques are explored later in this book.

Other approaches from the humanistic school include: Eric Berne's Transactional Analysis and Fritz Perl's Gestalt Therapy. Persons interested in these approaches are directed to the further reading provided at the end of this book. Persons interested in training to develop their counselling skills are advised to contact the British Association of Counselling and Psychotherapy (BACP), whose address is provided at the back of this book.

> 'There are two ways of spreading light: to be the candle or the mirror that reflects it.'
>
> Edith Wharton

Integrative therapy

This type of therapy integrates and combines some of the ideas and working styles from the psychodynamic, cognitive and humanistic schools and works with the appropriate methods to suit the client, the time-frame of the therapy and the presenting issues. This can be seen as an advantage, although different therapists will have their own preferred models from each paradigm and may have a bias towards these. Critics of this approach argue that therapists working in this way may not cover specific theories in sufficient depth to work with them effectively. An alternative perspective would be that any therapist working to an ethical framework would take responsibility for their learning and professional development and seek further training to update their knowledge and skills.

Planning worry time, writing hassle lists and creating possibilities

If you feel overwhelmed by worries and they create a burden to daily living, it is wise to plan a set time each week or maybe even each day to just sit and worry! Experience all the worries in one go, write them down, be aware of them and then be free to move along with other things without these burdens being carried around every moment of every day. Let yourself have worry-free time as well.

You can make use of your worry time to become more aware of personal stress by writing down all the things that hassle you and make a note of which can be changed and which cannot and which are most important to you. It is surprising how many can actually be changed if you put your mind to it.

Hassles

Write a list of all the things that hassle you.

Make a note of which you can change and which you cannot, and what things you would like to change.

Take one hassle at a time and write a second list of all the possible things you could do to change or manage this. The techniques explored throughout this book provide some possible strategies. Be imaginative and free when you think of all the possible strategies; let your mind be really creative.

'Possibility is the seed of the flower.'

Richard Wilkins

You can discuss your list of possibilities with friends or family to gather other perspectives. Once you have a list of all the possibilities, scan through it and see which ideas appeal and which do not. Commit to making the changes that appeal to you step by step. Sometimes you may need to change the situation, other times you can work on other strategies to build your coping resources and self management.

Letting go of control

Often our stress can be linked to a need to control things and people and for them to be how we think they should be to meet our own needs, wants and demands. Some situations in life cannot be changed, some things in life just are as they are. It is our resistance that can contribute to our stress. For example: getting stuck in a traffic jam on the way to work; missing a train; standing in a queue at the bank; receiving poor service in a restaurant;

Example of possibilities

Goal: to give up smoking (used as a method of coping with stress)

Learn relaxation techniques
Learn breathing techniques
Start an exercise session
Go for a walk instead of having a cigarette
Attend a smoking cessation course
Use nicotine replacement (patches, gum, plastic cigarette)
Smoke herbal cigarettes
Avoid places where people smoke
Go cold turkey
Cut down by 1 a day
Don't smoke before 11am or after 8pm
Take 10 deep breaths before having a cigarette
Change brands or smoke roll-ups
Put cigarettes out of reach
Buy fewer cigarettes
Save money
Put all smoked cigarettes into a glass of water and observe how dirty the water becomes

Aim to include all possibilities on the list. The person can then decide which ones would work most effectively for them.

being delayed at the airport. These situations can feel inconvenient and troublesome. Maintaining the internal conflict throughout the experience just adds to the discomfort we feel. Prolonging the experience by allowing it to become the focus of the whole day adds to our discomfort and makes it even more painful and disruptive.

Focusing on everything we think is wrong prevents us from seeing what is right and what can be appreciated. Focusing on poor service in a restaurant prevents us from enjoying the company we are with and even the food we are eating. Focusing on being stuck in a traffic jam prevents us from appreciating that we are fortunate to have a car; focusing on being stuck at the airport prevents us from looking forward to the fact that we have ahead of us a holiday or that we have just experienced a holiday.

> 'Don't sweat the small stuff... and it's all small stuff'
>
> Richard Carlson (1997)

Letting go of the need to control everything and everyone gives us the freedom to choose to make the most of what is. It can free us from the mental constraint of having to have everything happen a specific way. Of course, it is pleasant to get all the things we want and for everything to happen as we would want it to happen all the time. Sometimes, there can be a greater purpose for things happening that create our resistance; maybe we have something to learn from the experience that will enhance our personal growth. Maybe something better will come from an experience.

Letting go of the need to control can help us to make the internal changes we need to move forward. Complaining that our partner doesn't do this or do that is fairly futile and creates disruption in the relationship; it doesn't help us to value what they add to our lives. Complaining that our boss won't give us a pay rise doesn't assist with improving our circumstances. It doesn't help us to move towards making steps and changes to get what we want. Complaining that we don't have time to exercise doesn't help us to find solutions to manage our time. These things just add to our unhappiness and can prevent us from seeing that we have a choice and that we can make changes if we want to. If our partner doesn't take us out, what stops us from planning our own social events? If our boss won't give us a pay rise, what stops us from changing jobs? If we don't make time for ourselves to exercise, who can?

We can blame the events of our life and how we feel on external forces. We can blame ourselves, our lack of self-discipline, our lack of willpower, our unattractiveness, our lack of confidence, our lack of qualifications and so on. Alternatively, we can take back our power and make changes internally (how we think and feel) or externally (by changing the situation) and take responsibility for ourselves to move forward with our lives and create a new story and experience.

> 'The power is within you.'
>
> Louise Hay

Saying YES

A fairly natural response to stressful and uncomfortable events is to wonder 'why me?' and 'why now?' Losing a job, ending a relationship or having to meet a tight deadline at work or for a study course can lead us to feel overwhelmed and sorry for ourselves. Occasionally it is good and very necessary to have fleeting moments of self-pity and give ourselves some time out from stress and dealing with what is happening. However, staying in a cycle of self-pity and not dealing with it will not help to improve things. It will most likely lower our self-esteem and make us feel worse, which could have a further negative impact on our situation.

> 'If you look at everything you like in your life, you'll find that you had something to do with getting it — even if it was the passive act of allowing it to happen.'
>
> John Roger and Peter McWilliams
> (You Can't Afford the Luxury of a Negative Thought)

At some point we need to acknowledge what is happening and start making plans to improve things, take action and make one small step forward at a time. Saying YES is the first step to accepting responsibility and making the decision to move forward. It is acknowledging what is present and making the commitment to deal with what is happening and exploring the learning from the event.

> 'I only have "yes" men around me. Who needs "no" men?'
>
> Mae West

It may not always be possible to change life events and situations, but we can change how we respond. All the techniques explored in Part Two are ways of making a first step towards managing the physical, behavioural, mental and emotional signs and symptoms of stress and making a forward movement in ourselves and our lives.

Stress management affirmation

Repeat the following affirmation as often as possible to help with responsibility and self-belief:

'Yes, I can handle this...'

Managing fear and comfort zones

Fear plays an important role in stress management. The key learning for anyone who wants to make changes in their life is that change can be scary. One thing is for sure, the scariness or fear never goes away; it is an emotion that is always present (as are all emotions), so the priority is how we manage it

> 'No man is a failure who is enjoying life.'
>
> William Feather

and whether we allow it to rule us or whether we allow ourselves to manage it.

A brilliant starting point for anyone interested in making changes and managing fear is to read the book or listen to the tape of the book *Feel the Fear and Do It Anyway* by Susan Jeffers. This is a really motivational and inspirational book about how to manage fear and the change process.

One strategy for helping to overcome fear is to do things that move you slightly out of your comfort zone. This provides a challenge but, when you succeed at it, it feels great. A simple example for all trainee exercise teachers may be the first time they stand up and teach in front of a group of people. Most will feel some fear and discomfort, but once you do it, you have pushed your comfort zone a little. Adding constant stretches to your comfort zone can be a real confidence boost. The key is making one small step at a time. For example, the first movement out of a comfort zone for some trainee exercise teachers may be phoning for information on the study course; the

Expanding comfort zones

Think about 10 things you would like to do but are a little scared of doing and do them one at a time. Examples may include:
Travelling abroad for a holiday on your own.
Asking someone out on a date.
Taking a study course.
Teaching your first exercise class.

The key is to start small, learn from all experiences and not give up. If the first attempt fails, keep working towards what you want to achieve.

next discomfort may be booking a place; the next step, receiving the information pack; then attending on the first day, and so on. Each step is a step out of one's comfort zone and towards being an exercise instructor.

Creative work

How can creativity help with stress?

We are by nature creative beings and the energy that our creative self has within can be tremendous! Utilising this energy to express our inner feelings, thoughts and tensions is often very useful and empowering. Channelling this energy constructively is far healthier than storing it inwardly to create disharmony and tension.

'Risk'

To laugh is to risk appearing the fool
To weep is to risk appearing sentimental
To reach out is to risk involvement
To expose feelings is to risk exposing your true self
To place your ideas and dreams before the crowd is to risk their love
To love is to risk not being loved in return
To live is to risk dying
To hope is to risk despair
To try is to risk failure
But the greatest hazard in life is to risk nothing
The one who risks nothing does nothing and has nothing – and finally is nothing
He may avoid sufferings and sorrow,
But he simply cannot learn, feel, change, grow or love
Chained by his certitude, he is a slave; he has forfeited freedom
Only one who risks is free!

Author unknown.

Stress and tension are often linked with an unrecognised or unexpressed emotion. Creativity can be a safe and easy method to explore feelings such as anger, grief, guilt, fear or frustration in a transformative way. Some common reactions to releasing an emotion and seeing it stare back at you on the paper are, for example, 'I never knew I was holding that much angry tension inside' or 'I can't believe I was storing that much grief' and many times people feel the tension just flow from their whole self as the creative process unfolds.

'If I had to define life in a word, it would be: life is creation'.

Claude Bernard

Creative work can help to:

- identify stressful, or otherwise difficult-to-express feelings and thoughts
- release these stressful or difficult-to-express feelings and thoughts
- promote personal growth and insight
- assist with problem solving
- integrate the mental and emotional aspects of ourselves.

Creativity is often an untapped resource for releasing stress and pent-up emotions. Many people will dismiss creative methods and say 'I can't draw', 'I'm not artistic' or 'It feels alien or childlike'. In fact, childhood seems to be where our creative bud is quashed and many people feel reluctant to try again with this innate form of expression.

Throughout our daily lives, both consciously and unconsciously, we absorb and cram our minds with images, words, symbols, sounds and sensations, which can in times of stress become distorted and invasive. For example, we may say 'I can't bear that loud music right now', or 'I just can't think in this cluttered environment', or 'I feel like my head is going to explode', or 'I feel so wound up'. When we try to sleep, we may be confronted with a busy mind that won't switch off from the thoughts, chatter, images of the day/week and so on. At times of stress this can be overwhelming.

Tapping into the chaos and negative thoughts and feelings through creative work is one way or step towards feeling more relaxed and in harmony with the self. It can be literally like emptying a rubbish bin that has become full up. Creative expression can help to clear out the old thoughts and feelings and make space for new and fresh thoughts and feelings.

How to begin

While the product of expression is important, we must remember that the process of creation is what is profoundly transformative. Ideally, don't try to conform to any preconceived ideas about how your images should look and don't let the inner critical voice thwart your efforts, although acknowledgement of these aspects of the self can sometimes be equally useful in understanding your personal process.

Let your hands, fingers, brushes, crayons or other tools go where they want to. It may be that using your less dominant hand will release your innate creative flow more easily. Don't be afraid of experimenting with either or both hands, just go with what feels right for you at the time. Some suggestions on how you may want to begin exploring your creative self are:

Doodles

Materials:

- Large sheet of plain paper/lining paper
- Selection of coloured markers/pens/pastels/ pencils
- Masking tape to fix paper to a table or floor

Process: Choose a quiet undisturbed space and time. Secure a large sheet of paper with masking tape to an appropriate surface. Select marker/pen/pastel/pencil of your choice and, with eyes open or shut, whichever feels right at the time, start doodling on the paper. Stop when it feels right. Stand back and absorb what has emerged. Add to it if you want to with more of the same or maybe you want to add words or a title to it. This only takes a few minutes and you can repeat it as often as your mood takes you.

Painting your picture

Materials:

- Selection of coloured paints (acrylics are versatile and quick-drying)
- Brushes, palette knife and/or your fingers
- Wet/dry palette or plate to put paints on
- Canvas board/s in your choice of size

Process: Give yourself a time and place where you will not be disturbed or interrupted. Using brushes, tools or fingers, build up an expression of colours, textures, shapes and forms that flow from you onto the canvas board. There are no rigid guidelines, except *do not censor* what comes out; just let your picture do its own thing and build up by itself. Feel free to experiment with your less dominant hand.

It may not seem to take on any form or structure until you have finished, when, as you stand back and see your creation, it speaks to you of a feeling or situation. If a title or words come to mind note them, if not don't worry. Delight in what your creative self has produced and derive any meaning it has for you at the time. Take note of what the colours are saying about how you feel – maybe you have used lots of red and this represents anger to you or maybe lots of black evokes the feelings of wanting to hide at this time. Again the meanings are for you to interpret. If an emotional reaction floods over you, again let it flow. Let out the tension.

Collage creation

Materials:

- Selection of any items you have to hand such as magazines, newspapers, feathers, glitter, beads, twigs, leaves or catalogues
- Scissors
- Glue
- Large sheet of paper or stiff card

Process: Go with whatever your creative self wants to do. It may be that you want to build a free-form collage by building images and pieces which layer and form in an abstract way. Perhaps you want to have a theme like '*This is me*' or '*This is how I feel*' and pick images, words and colours to represent aspects of your mood, feelings or situation. The only point I want to reiterate with this process, as with all creative projects, is *do not censor*. Alternatively, you may not discover exactly how you feel consciously until your collage conveys this to you in some way when it is finished. Feel free to explore words or stories that go with your creation and see where they take you on your journey of discovery.

Sculpture your vulture

Material:

- Modelling clay

Process: Choose an appropriate space and time where you will be undisturbed and are comfortable. Let your creative self mould and shape the clay into expressions of the moment. Do not have any preconceived ideas but just let your feelings and tension sink into the clay and image. If, for example, anger is your particular difficult emotion, perhaps you could sculpt a creature that represents that emotion. You may be surprised at what your creative self reveals. Respect the process even if your piece ends up in your eyes as an ugly vulture – look at what part of you needs to express and release and appreciate that aspect of yourself.

A journal of discovery

Writing out thoughts and feelings in the form of a journal is another method for getting to know how you think and feel. It is also a method of releasing pent-up feelings and emotions in a safe way. The key is to reserve any judgement of the thoughts and feelings identified, and just recognise them. These can be reviewed alone or, ideally, explored with a good friend who can help strategise to find a variety of ways for improving events by taking specific actions such as managing time, exercising, delegating tasks, asking for support at work and so on.

Materials:

- A blank book/diary of your choice
- Pen/coloured pens/images of your choice

Process: Choose a time and place where you will not be disturbed. Experiment with writing in your book in different places such as the park, beach, garden or café. Write as often as you can. This may not be every day but two or three times a week. If you are feeling particularly stressed or tense it might suit you to release your feelings into the book more often, but again it is up to you to find your own pace.

Let this be a personal expression of your thoughts, feelings, fantasies and dreams. Unless you choose to share these with others, keep it somewhere where it will remain safe and confidential. If you find your inner critic prevents you from writing freely, focus on those critical messages and write about them. These may help you to see where blocks are and much learning or movement can be experienced as a result.

If you feel able to doodle and draw or stick images in alongside your words, then this too will add to your creative self being acknowledged and consequently a release of stressful/difficult emotions/thoughts often happens.

Don't try to organise or structure your

writing – if it seems chaotic or confusing, accept this as part of how you're experiencing your inner and outer world right now. Similarly, do not try to edit or correct spellings or punctuation, just write as it flows in its raw, uncensored way from your creative self.

You may discover there is a rhythm or rhyme emerging in your words of expression and it may be that you would like to work these into a poem as an option.

Remember to write about the positive experiences and feelings too, as often we tend to focus just on the negatives. Again, much learning, growth and release can occur when we give ourselves permission to experience the emotion of *joy*.

Sounding out

Our voice is the meeting place where our mind and body join together to express. Our vocal chords are the channel and link that connect these two aspects of ourselves. Our culture tends to discourage using our voices in any manner other than to talk or sing. There are not many outlets for uninhibited sounding. Often as children we are told, 'Keep quiet' or 'Don't make a sound'. So there are many reminders of keeping our voices down that stifle self-expression. As adults, often the joyous noises from lovemaking are tempered or muffled, so as to not let anyone hear how much we are enjoying ourselves.

Making sounds is a big part of self-expression. You only have to think of the times that, at the soonest opportunity it is safe to do so, we let out long, heavy sighs of frustration or stress. It is as if our bodies just have to let us and others know how we are feeling by letting off steam. Or the familiar *Aahhrrr* response if a situation or person triggers our feelings of anger and rage.

Given the chance not to be heard by others, often we do let out stress, joy and frustration while safely behind the wheel of a car. Here it is soundproofed, private and secure and we can let out feelings and expression. Some alternative suggestions to explore this natural way of expression and tension release, either alone or with someone with whom you feel comfortable, might be:

Process

- In any large open space where you are unlikely to meet with others to inhibit or disturb you in your process, such as a wood or forest, explore and let out any sounds that come forth as loudly and for as long as you feel able. Certain vibrations and resonances will feel more in tune to you than others. If working with another person it might be useful to sound back what they are sounding out and then swap and repeat the process as many times as feels right. Just explore and release what comes naturally. You may have words or phrases that want to be aired, and if this occurs just go with the flow.

- In the privacy of your own home maybe you have a favourite song or background music that is conducive to releasing some sounds, words or songs. If you wish to move and dance at the same time then let your body move in the way it wants to. It is important to not worry about being in tune or in time, just go with your natural form of expression.

- You may find using a tape recorder useful, in that playing back to yourself the sounds you make can release some powerful feelings and aid stress release.

- Try using percussion instruments, even home-made ones, to aid the creative process. Sometimes an instrument can articulate more easily a sound or feeling we have difficulty in expressing. If you find a sound that speaks your feelings then repeat it as often as you need, with or without your own voice alongside it.

Smooth moves

Movement can be another area in which to explore the creative self. Apart from specific exercises, dancing or sexual activity, it is generally an untapped area of expression. Our bodies store tension and stress and we often complain of the physical sensations that this tension creates within us. Movement of our bodies can be a very powerful way of tapping into some feelings and bringing release.

Here are some exercises that you may wish to try either alone or with some others you are comfortable with.

Dancing with your shadow: Place a bright lamp/light on the floor of a dark room where there is a blank wall on which you can project your shadow. Use music if you want and try not to let self-criticism impede your flow and movement. Allow your instincts to roam and move as your mood and body explore shapes and shadows on the wall. It may seem quite strange at first to see your body shadow reflected and distorted as you move and turn, but stay with it and see what unfolds.

Tune into your inner experience and if you feel that quick, jerky movements are to the fore one moment then slow smooth glides the next, just allow this to happen.

Free form: You may wish to move in free form with your eyes closed. It may be helpful to have someone you trust with you to guide and keep you from bumping into things. This often heightens awareness of your body and inner world as the focus of the outside diminishes. Follow your impulses and try not to let your preconceived ideas or your inner critic get in the way of your creative self. Enjoy the experience and see where it takes you.

Remember our expression is ours to interpret, it is not for others to give meaning to. While the product of expression is important, remember that the process of creation is what is profoundly transformative.

Letters or lyrics

Another method of releasing emotions is to write out feelings in a letter and then burn the letter. This can be very cathartic! It may also be a little scary for some people. The key is to withhold any judgement you may have about yourself for thinking these thoughts or having these feelings, and just let them out and release them safely. If emotions are allowed to build up they tend to find a way of popping out in some guise. This may be through illness (physical/medical) or through addictive habits (behavioural) or problems in relationships (social) and so on.

Emotions and thoughts need to be set free to make space for fresh emotions and thoughts. Songwriters express their innermost feelings in their lyrics and we can all associate with some lyrics in certain songs. We may not be famous songwriters but we can still express our internal struggles and joys.

Creature comforts

There are numerous simple activities that we can fit into our life that bring comfort when we are stressed. The key is to recognise the things that bring you comfort, and help you to relax and unwind. The things we find relaxing will vary from one individual to another, the secret is to find something that makes us feel good.

> **Stress relief**
>
> Make a list of your own creature comforts and start planning time for these. You can use the list below if you feel too stressed to think about these.
>
> If you are in the middle of experiencing a stressful event, make time for one or more of these.

Creature comfort list

Hot, fragrant, bubble bath in candlelight with soft music

Writing a letter to or telephoning a friend

Massage and aromatherapy

Hot shower

Curling up on the sofa with a video

Reading the papers in bed on a Sunday morning

Sofa and a face pack

Going for a manicure and pedicure

Going horse-riding in the countryside

Spending a day at a health spa

Yoga class

Watching a feel-good film

Cuddling up with my kids

Daydreaming about my friends and how they are to stop me focusing on my stuff and smiling and being grateful for them all because I know I am not on my own

Walking on the beach

Reading a magazine

Reading chick literature

Dancing to a piece of music

Pruning my roses with a glass of red wine (NB: Pruning scissors work better than red wine!)

Making love with my partner

Daydreaming anywhere peaceful, letting my thoughts come and go, and fantasising

Visualising the gardens at a country retreat I visit

Cuddling up with my teddy and letting myself feel sorry for myself and have time out

Going for a walk with my partner

Listening to music by candlelight

Sleeping

Drawing pictures

Writing essays

Travelling away for the weekend

Going clothes shopping

Driving in the city at night (NYC)

Going to the gym

Booking a short break or holiday, so I have something to look forward to

Drinking a cup of hot chocolate

As a mum, I'd say going to bed early with hot chocolate and a movie

Driving to a place with great scenic views, no cars, no people, and no phones and walking my dog, with a flask of tea and snacks, and having a me-time picnic!

Going for a run

Sitting in a coffee shop and watching the world rush by, instead of me!

Watching a funny movie and having a beer

Thanks to all the wonderful people who contributed their personal creature comforts to develop this list.

STRATEGIES FOR MANAGING THE PHYSICAL AND BEHAVIOURAL SIGNS AND SYMPTOMS OF STRESS

5

In order to manage the physical and behavioural signs and symptoms of stress, we need to be aware of what signs and symptoms we have developed that may be linked to stress. Table 5.1 provides a checklist for identifying some of the physical and behavioural signs and symptoms of stress.

What techniques are available to manage the physical and behavioural signs and symptoms of stress?

There are many ways to combat the signs and symptoms of stress on a physical and behavioural level, including:

- posture awareness exercises
- breathing exercises
- rest, relaxation and meditation exercises
- diet and nutrition
- other lifestyle and behaviour changes (smoking, alcohol)
- desk mobility exercises.

Physical activity and exercise are explored in the next chapter.

Posture awareness

Why is correct posture important?

Postural misalignment can affect the functioning of our inner organs, for example allowing the mid-section to rest continuously in a slumped position can affect the movement of the diaphragm muscle that assists with breathing. Poor posture that is maintained and uncorrected for long periods of time can also lead to permanent postural problems, for example hunched back (kyphosis), which can contribute to the risk of falls in later life, or hollow back (lordosis), which can contribute to back pain. Prolonged muscle imbalance caused by holding an incorrect posture will also lead to increased muscle tension and tightness in some muscles and a lack of strength in the opposing muscles.

Exercises to open and align posture can help to alleviate a build-up of muscular tension, and can also enhance the functioning of the inner organs

Posture awareness activity

How are you sitting right now? Stay in that position.

Become aware of the position of your shoulders, neck, abdominals, feet, legs and arms. Notice your thoughts and notice how you feel. Now change your posture and sit more upright and open. Again, notice how your postural change affects your inner thoughts and feelings.

Be aware of how you position your body throughout the day to promote further awareness, which can help towards developing better habits.

Use the posture awareness exercises below to correct your posture.

Table 5.1	The physical and behavioural signs and symptoms checklist		
Physical		**Behavioural**	
Spots		Eating more or less	
Shoulder tension		Drinking more stimulants	
Skin disorders		Smoking more	
Chest pain		Swearing	
Increased heart rate		Argumentative, aggressive behaviour (violence or crime)	
Nervous indigestion		Crying	
Fast, shallow breathing			
Upper back hunched		Increased or decreased sexual libido	
Yawning or sighing a lot		Excessive talking	
Increased blood pressure		Rapid eye movements	
Abdominal pain		Foot-tapping	
Sexual difficulties		Inability to sit still	
Clenched jaw		Picking at skin	
Menstrual disorders		Grinding teeth	
Flatulence		Gripping hands	
Allergies		Nervous laughter	
Hair loss		Driving faster	
Dry mouth		Exercising more or less	
Tense forehead/headaches			

(for example the diaphragm). Standing and moving with correct posture also gives the impression of greater confidence and walking with upright posture can increase personal confidence. Open posture is expansive. Hunched-over posture gives the appearance of closing in on oneself.

Posture awareness exercise 1: Standing posture

- Stand with feet hip-width apart
- Keep feet parallel
- Distribute weight between heel-bone, big toe and little toe (three-point weight distribution)

- Spread toes
- Align second toe with knee and hip
- Find neutral pelvic position (public bone and hip-bones in line to ensure no or minimal forward or backward tilt of pelvis)
- Lengthen torso and neck
- Tighten the deeper abdominal muscles (so that the contraction can be maintained)
- Look forwards – chin parallel to floor
- Shoulders to be relaxed and down
- Squeeze shoulder blades down
- Place hands by sides, palms facing forwards

Posture awareness exercise 2: Seated posture

- Sit on a chair with buttocks on the front third of the chair
- Align knees with ankles
- Feet to be hip-width apart
- Keep feet parallel
- Distribute weight evenly between heel-bone, big toe and little toe (three-point weight distribution)
- Spread toes
- Sit upright and lengthen spine
- Lift out of sitting bones to find neutral pelvic position (keep public bone and hip-bones in line to ensure no or minimal forward or backward tilt of pelvis)
- Lengthen torso and neck
- Tighten the abdominals (so that the contraction can be maintained)
- Look forwards – keep chin parallel to floor
- Shoulders to be relaxed and down
- Squeeze shoulder blades down
- Place hands by the side of chair, palms facing forwards

Instant stress relief

Stop what you are doing right now.

Open up your posture as described above.

Notice how much better it feels to lengthen your spine and open up your posture.

Breathing awareness

Why is correct breathing important?

There is a tendency towards shallow and rapid breathing, using the upper thoracic or chest to breathe (where the upper chest and shoulders lift and lower as we breathe). This is a particular pattern among people who are very tense and stressed, and also among people who are sedentary. Poor breathing habits such as these can contribute to anxiety and panic.

Ideally, we should use the whole of the ribcage and abdomen when we breathe (diaphragm and abdominal breathing). Focusing on deeper and slower breathing can help to reduce the immediate and long-term effects of the fight and flight response and can help return the body to a more natural unstressed state. It will allow more oxygen to be circulated into the bloodstream and facilitate the removal of carbon dioxide, thus allowing more oxygen to reach the brain, which can encourage the release of endorphins (the feel-good hormone).

Breathing awareness exercise

Start by finding an open posture position (seated, lying or standing). Focus awareness on the depth, speed and feeling of the breath. The eyes can be closed or can focus on a specific

Breathing awareness activity

How are you breathing right now?

Does your abdomen rise and fall as you breathe? Do you feel relaxed?

Try lying on the floor with one hand on your chest and the other hand on your abdomen.

Notice which hand moves higher and whether there are any restrictions to your breathing.

Use the breathing awareness exercise to enhance breathing.

spot looking forwards or slightly downwards (make sure the posture position doesn't change).

- Take the breath slightly deeper into the lower ribcage (most people take very shallow breaths into the upper chest area only).
- Keep the breath soft, smooth and rhythmical
- Find a natural breathing pace.
- Find a natural breathing power (not forcing or straining).
- Let the breath become effortless and allow it to flow freely.
- Notice the abdomen rise and fall.
- Allow the breath to quieten and calm the mind.
- Allow a few minutes just to focus on the breathing and stillness.

Instant stress relief

Stop what you are doing right now.

Take 10 deep slow breaths and notice how your body relaxes.

Breathe in for a count of four, hold for a count of four, and breathe out slowly for a count of eight.

Focus on breathing more slowly and deeply and listening to the sound of your breathing.

Relaxation awareness

Why is relaxation important?

Constant hurrying without finding time to relax places the body and mind under incredible stress. Both need time out to rest and be still. Without appropriate relaxation there can be a tendency to seek other ways of unwinding, such as drinking alcohol, smoking and so on. These substances do provide a short-term fix to manage stress, but if used constantly as stress relievers will have their own impact on health. This will be explored a little further later in this chapter.

Time for relaxation allows the body to be still and provides a healthier alternative to provide rest for the body. Relaxation can provide physical release for the muscles and joints and other bodily systems. It can also bring a stillness to the mind, allowing it to become less fogged, so that clarity of thinking can return.

Relaxation exercises can be performed in any position that feels comfortable. The most common positions used, which help to maintain an open posture, are described next.

Relaxation postures/poses

Ex 5.1a	**Relaxation posture: Sitting pose**

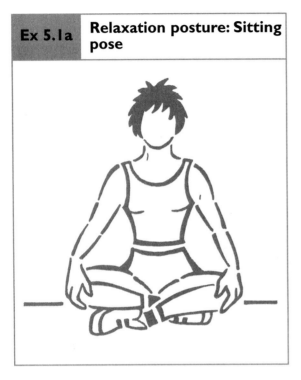

Purpose

Opens the hips and strengthens the back and core muscles. Prepares for meditation and awareness of the mind.

Starting position and instructions

- Sit with the legs crossed one in front of the other, in line with the pubic bone.
- Sit fully onto the sitting bones.
- Lengthen the spine and relax the shoulders.
- Position the hands either: on the lap with one palm up resting on top of the other palm, arms relaxed; or one hand resting on each knee.

Teaching points

- Maintain a neutral pelvic position.
- Draw the abdominal muscles in slightly.
- Breathe naturally.
- Alternate the leg that is in front (each time you sit in this position) to ensure equal opening of the hips.

Adaptations

- Sit against a wall to support the spine.
- Sit in a chair with the feet firmly on the floor and the spine lengthened.

Ex 5.1b	Relaxation posture: Lying (corpse) pose

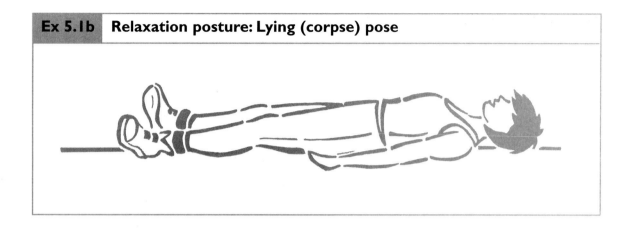

Purpose

Promotes relaxation of the body and focuses the attention of the mind on the body in preparation for meditation.

Starting position and instructions

- Lie on your back with legs straight, arms at the side of the body and palms facing upwards.
- Lengthen the neck and draw the shoulders away from the ears.
- Relax the hips and lower back.
- Relax the legs and allow the feet to roll outwards.

Teaching points

- Notice how the body contacts the floor.
- Become aware of the body, where tension is stored, where there is tightness – allow the body to let go and to relax.
- Allow the breath to become deeper and softer, effortless.
- Allow the mind to feel peaceful.

Adaptation

Lie in any position that feels comfortable. However, corpse position allows the body to be most open.

Ex 5.1c	**Relaxation posture: Chair seated pose**

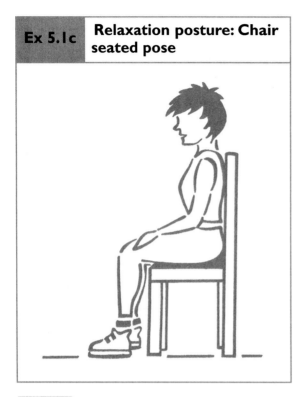

Purpose

Strengthens the back and core muscles. Grounds the feet to the floor and prepares for meditation and awareness of the mind.

Starting position and instructions

- Sit on a chair with the feet firmly on the floor.
- Shuffle the buttocks back so that the sitting bones press back into the chair.
- Allow the back to rest back and be supported by the chair.
- Lengthen the spine and relax the shoulders.
- Position the hands either: on the lap with one palm up resting on top of the other palm, arms relaxed; or one hand resting on each knee.

Teaching points

- Maintain a neutral pelvic position.
- Draw the abdominal muscles in lightly towards the spine.
- Breathe naturally.

Adaptations

- Sit without the back resting at the back of the chair to increase the work of the core muscles, open the posture and make the relaxation more conscious (less likely to fall asleep).
- Use the floor seated or lying positions.

Preparing for and ending a relaxation exercise

Preparing to start relaxation

- Ensure you are in a quiet space that will be free from distraction and interruptions for the desired period (turn off mobile phones etc.).
- Select one of the relaxation scripts on pages 65–72 (the scripts can be memorised, taped or read by another person).
- Select one of the relaxation postures on pages 62–4 or another position that feels comfortable to lie in, so that the body is supported and the posture open.
- Make sure you are warm and comfortable (pillow and blankets, lights off, candlelight if necessary and appropriate).
- Settle into the position and allow time to be still.
- Be aware of any external noise and distraction and then focus away from these.
- Focus inward and on how you are breathing (see breathing exercise guidelines).
- Commence relaxation or short meditation.

Preparing to end relaxation

- Bring the mind's attention back to the room and notice the sounds you hear around you.
- Gently move toes and feet.
- Feel the energy move through your legs.
- Gently move fingers and hands.
- Feel the energy move through your arms.
- Gently move your head from the right side to the left.
- Feel the energy move through your head.

If in a lying posture:

- Bend your knees and place your feet on the floor.
- Allow your legs to bend over towards the right; hold for 10 seconds.
- Return legs to centre and allow them to lower to the left; hold for 10 seconds.
- Return legs to centre.
- Hug knees to chest and curl head towards knees.
- In your own time, roll onto one side and gradually raise your body to a standing position.
- Shake out the whole body slowly and steadily.

If in a seated posture:

- In your own time, gradually raise your body to a standing position.
- Shake out the whole body slowly and steadily.

Relaxation techniques and scripts

Active muscular relaxation

Active muscular relaxation involves following instructions to actively tighten, extend or move different parts of the body and then allow them to relax and be still.

Advantages: It is a useful technique for people initially learning to relax as it is a fairly simple method to learn and can raise body awareness. This can be a particularly important skill to learn for persons who lack body awareness and carry a lot of tension in their body posture. It can help them to find active ways of releasing some of that tension. It also has the advantage that it requires little imagination.

Disadvantages: Individuals with low body awareness may find it difficult to isolate different body parts when they first use this technique. The technique is also inappropriate for persons with injuries or certain physical disabilities. A further disadvantage is that tensing the body part prior to releasing tension may actually increase tension and make it harder to relax.

Active muscular relaxation script

- Sit or lie in a comfortable position (see relaxation and meditation postures on pages 62–4).
- Allow your body to relax and lengthen.
- Allow the muscles to soften.
- Focus your awareness on your breathing.
- Notice the depth and pace of your breathing.
- Allow your breath to become slower, softer and deeper.
- Take your mind's awareness to your body, starting with the feet.
- Spread and separate your toes, feeling the tension in the feet.
- Flex your toes towards your knees, feeling the tension in the lower leg.
- Stay aware of the tension; breathe steadily in and out.
- Then let the toes and feet relax, letting go of any tension in the lower legs.
- Be still and breathe softly and deeply.
- Take your mind's awareness to the thigh muscles.
- Allow the muscles at the front of the thigh to tighten without locking the knee.
- Tighten the muscles at the back of the thigh.
- Squeeze the buttocks tight.
- Stay aware of the tension in the thighs and buttocks; breathe steadily in and out.
- Then let the thigh and buttock muscles relax.
- Feel the hip joint open and soften.
- Feel the whole of the legs relax and soften.
- Be still and breathe softly and deeply.
- Focus your mind's awareness on the abdomen.
- Draw the abdominal muscles in tightly towards your backbone.
- Feel the sides of the abdomen draw in tight.
- Feel the muscles of the lower back tighten.
- Stay aware of the tension; experience the feeling of a corset tightening around the centre of the body; breathe steadily in and out.
- Then release the tension in these muscles, feel the centre of the body relax and let go.
- Be still and breathe softly and deeply.
- Focus your mind's awareness on the shoulders and upper back.
- Squeeze the shoulders towards the ears.
- Feel the tension increase in the muscles of the upper back and the back of the neck, breathe steadily in and out.
- Then allow the muscles to let go and release.
- Lengthen the ears away from the shoulders.
- Feel the chin tucking towards the body.
- Feel the muscles in between the shoulder blades drawing downwards and tightening.
- Stay aware of the tension; breathe steadily in and out.
- Then release the tension in these muscles, allowing the body to let go.
- Be still and breathe softly and deeply.
- Focus your awareness on the muscles of the arms.
- Extend the arms and tense all the muscles in the upper and lower arms; breathe steadily in and out.
- Clench the fists to increase the tension.
- Stay aware of the tension, breathing steadily in and out.
- Then allow the muscles to release and let go.
- Spread the fingers and open up the hands.
- Extend the fingers as far away from the shoulders as you can.
- Stay aware of the tension in the muscles of the hands and arms; breathe steadily in and out.
- Then release and let go and allow the arms to soften and relax.
- Allow the body to be still; breathe slowly and deeply.
- Focus your mind's awareness on the face and head.
- Open your mouth wide and feel the tension around the mouth and jaw.
- Stay aware of the tension; breathe steadily in and out.

- Then release and let go; allow the jaw to relax and wiggle the jaw a little.
- Stick out your tongue, then allow it to relax back into your mouth.
- Feel the tongue soften and the mouth and jaw relax; breathe steadily in and out.
- Wiggle your nose and then release.
- Feel the eye sockets opening and then release.
- Move the muscles in the forehead, then allow them to soften and relax.
- Let the body sink deeper and relax further.
- Feel any tension just easing away.
- Tighten the whole body one last time, extending your head and toes and fingers as far away from each other as you can.
- Release and let go; allow yourself to sigh.
- Take your mind's awareness back to your breathing.
- Focus on slower, deeper breathing.
- Allow your body to be still and silent.
- With every breath allow the body to relax further.
- Allow a feeling of relaxation and calm to spread through your whole body.

NB: Complete an ending to the relaxation here (see page 65).

Passive muscular relaxation

Passive muscular relaxation involves using the mind to focus on different body areas and using this awareness to relax each specific body part. There is no specific movement of any body part.

Advantage: Individuals who are able to focus and concentrate all their attention on their body will find this method very relaxing and calming. It is great for providing stillness to people who are very active. It is also a very effective method for people who have injuries or physical disabilities that make it uncomfortable or impossible to move specific body parts.

Disadvantage: This method may be frustrating for people who are very active and find it difficult to be still and relax. Individuals who find it difficult to focus may also struggle with the imagery of letting each different body part relax.

Passive muscular relaxation script

- Sit or lie in a comfortable position (see relaxation and meditation postures on pages 62–64).
- Allow your body to relax and lengthen.
- Allow the muscles to soften.
- Focus your awareness on your breathing.
- Notice the depth and pace of your breathing.
- Allow your breath to become slower, softer and deeper.
- Take your mind's awareness to your body, starting with the feet.
- Allow the feet to soften and relax; let go of any tension.
- Allow the ankle joints to open and relax.
- Feel the calf muscles and muscles at the front of the shin soften.
- Take a deeper breath and on the outward breath allow the lower leg to relax and soften even further.
- Take your mind's awareness to the knee joints.
- Allow the knee joints to open and relax.
- Feel the muscles at the front of the thigh soften.
- Feel the muscles at the back of the thigh lengthen and relax.
- Take a deeper breath and on the outward breath allow the whole of the legs to relax and let go.
- Focus your mind's awareness to the hip joints.
- Allow the hip joints to open up and relax.
- Feel the buttock muscles relax and soften.
- Feel the muscles around the hip release and open.

- Focus your mind's awareness on the spine.
- Start at the base of the spine and be mindful of each vertebra up to the skull.
- Feel each vertebra open up.
- Allow the muscles around the vertebrae (spine) to relax and lengthen.
- Allow all the tension to ease away.
- Allow the shoulder blades to separate and open up.
- Take a deep breath and allow the whole spine to lengthen and relax.
- Focus on the abdominal muscles.
- Allow them to release.
- Notice how the breath fills the abdominal area.
- Observe the abdomen rising and falling with each breath.
- Notice the ribcage and the breastbone.
- Feel the muscles around the ribs relax.
- Allow the breath to become slower and deeper.
- Allow the ribs and the breastbone to soften.
- Focus your awareness on the shoulder joint.
- Allow the shoulder joint to open up and relax.
- Feel the muscles of the upper arm lengthen and relax.
- Notice the elbow joint.
- Feel the elbow joint relaxing and opening.
- Feel the muscles of the forearm relax and soften.
- Notice the wrists and the hands.
- Allow the tension to ease away.
- Allow the fingers to curl open and the tension to float away.
- Focus your mind's awareness on the head.
- Allow each of the facial muscles to soften and relax.
- Feel the jaw relax.
- Feel the tongue soften.
- Feel the lips gently touching and forming a soft smile.
- Allow the cheekbones to relax.
- Notice the eye sockets relaxing.
- Allow the forehead to relax.

- Feel any tension just easing away.
- Feel your body soften.
- Allow your body to feel light and relaxed.
- Take your mind's awareness back to your breathing.
- Focus on slower, deeper breathing.
- With every breath allow the body to relax further.
- Allow a feeling of peace and calm to spread through your whole body.

Note: On completion of relaxation a silent period can be allowed for individual mindfulness/ meditation.

NB: Complete an ending of the relaxation exercise here (see page 65).

Visualisation/guided fantasy relaxation

This involves following instructions to visualise specific images, people, events or environments that create a relaxed physiological response. It can also be used to take an individual on a specific fantasy journey by following specific instructions.

People: If people are used in the visualisation, it is essential to guide the individual to a person who is still with them, who they love and trust and who is helpful towards them. The visualisation script can follow instructions such as: Notice that person, see what they are doing, notice what they are wearing, look at their face, recognise any good feelings you experience being in that person's company, hear their voice if they are speaking, notice what they are saying, their voice tone and so on. You can focus on a specific friend or a group of people you like to spend time with.

Events: If events are visualised, it is essential to use an event with positive associations and memories. The visualisation script can follow: remember an event where you felt incredibly happy, positive and confident. Notice the sounds, the people around you, what you can see, what you can hear, notice the positive feelings you have inside and so on.

Images: If objects are visualised, they must be objects that the person has positive associations with, such as a photograph or teddy bear.

Environments: If a specific environment is used for visualisation, it must be a place where the person has experienced a good feeling and feels safe. It could be a home environment, a favourite room, a country retreat, your garden and so on.

Advantages: People who are able to visualise the pictures positively will experience the relaxation effectively. Providing specific instructions on what aspects of a visualisation to focus on can develop this mental awareness. Instructions can be to identify: pictures (colour of leaves and flowers), sounds (noise of trees rustling, the wind blowing, birds singing), smells (of flowers, grass, the air), sensations (the heat of the sun, coolness of the wind) and can touch all the body senses within the visualisation/fantasy.

Disadvantages: Some people may have a negative physiological response to certain images. For example, a sunny beach and the sea can bring a positive response for one person and negative response for another, depending on their experience and the images their mind conjures up. Visualising people can bring up distressing memories if the person is no longer present in the individual's life. The visual images an individual conjures will very much be determined by their state of mind and experience and some care should be taken when using this method. This technique also takes time and can also evoke deeper feelings in some individuals. Some people may not enjoy the experience of having to using their imagination.

Visualisation/guided fantasy relaxation script

- Sit or lie in a comfortable position (see relaxation and meditation postures on pages 62–64).
- Allow your body to relax and lengthen.
- Allow the muscles to soften.
- Focus your awareness on your breathing.
- Notice the depth and pace of your breathing.
- Allow your breath to become slower, softer and deeper.
- Take your mind's awareness to your body, starting with the feet and moving slowly upwards through the body.
- If you feel any tension, just notice it, and on the outward breath send the message for that body part to relax.
- Let the body relax deeply and sink into the floor.
- Notice in your mind's eye a gate.
- Notice the height of the gate, and what it is made from.
- Walk slowly in your mind's eye towards the gate.
- Beyond the gate is a beautiful garden where you feel totally safe and secure.
- As you reach the gate, you see a lock and key. Notice the lock and key, what they look like and how they feel.
- Allow your mind's eye to let you unlock and open the gate.
- As the gate opens you notice the beautiful garden.
- Notice the flowers you see, their colours and their smells.
- Notice the gentle sounds you hear around you, birds singing, the wind blowing softly.
- Notice the blue sky and the comfortable warmth of the sun.
- Feel the warmth of the sun against your skin.
- Close the gate behind you and then return your mind's focus back to the garden.

- As you look into the garden you notice a tree.
- Notice the type of tree you see, the size of the tree, the colours of the leaves and the trunk.
- Notice the grass and flowers around the tree.
- In your mind's eye allow yourself to walk towards the tree.
- Notice the sounds of the grass rustling under your feet as you walk slowly towards the tree.
- When you reach the tree, let yourself sit down and rest peacefully, taking in the beauty of the garden and the peaceful surroundings through all your senses.
- Allow yourself five minutes to sit still and appreciate the garden and be at peace with yourself... (NB: if you are reading this script, allow participants to have silent time here. Tell them you will be silent and not speak for five minutes.) On completion of the five minutes continue the script.
- Now let yourself become aware of the sound of my voice again.
- Take one last look around you, and in your mind's eye look at the gate through which you entered the garden.
- Allow yourself to get up slowly, in your mind's eye, and walk steadily towards the gate.
- Notice the calm feelings you have from spending time in the garden.
- As you reach the gate, look around once more and notice the safety of the garden.
- Know that this is a place you can return to if you feel the need to retreat.
- Open the gate and walk though and then lock the gate after you.
- Walk away from the gate and prepare to bring your focus back into the room. Focus back on your breathing and awareness of your body.

NB: Complete an ending of the relaxation exercise here (see page 65).

Benson method of relaxation

This is an excellent method that can be used by individuals on their own and in their own time. It was developed by Herbert Benson for people with high blood pressure. He initially suggested that individuals sit still and quietly and focus on saying the word 'one' out loud on their outward breath for a short duration of time and just let the mind and body slow down with no specific effort.

The technique can be adapted in the following ways:

- The word 'one' can be replaced by other words that an individual may find more natural, such as calm, peace, love, still, silent, relax, ohm and so on.
- The word or mantra can be spoken silently within, rather than out loud.
- The technique can be used in everyday activities, for example when queuing at a supermarket, on the train, while out walking, at an office desk and so on.
- The technique can be used while sitting, standing or lying down and can easily be combined with other techniques.

Advantages: The greatest advantage is that the technique is very simple and is particularly beneficial for people who find it difficult to stop for long periods of time and just relax.

Disadvantages: This method may make some people feel a little self-conscious. Having to say a word or mantra out loud can be embarrassing. The alternative of saying the word or mantra inside without vocalising it will usually ease any embarrassment.

Adapted version of Benson method relaxation script

- Sit quietly with an open body posture.
- Focus on your breathing.
- As you breathe out, focus on a desired word (calm, one, peace, relax, joy).

- The word can be spoken out loud or quietly within.
- Practice this for about 5–10 minutes, just allowing the body to relax.

At the end of this technique it is worth noting how the experience felt. A notepad can be used to jot down thoughts and feelings that arose.

5-minute stress relief

Sit quietly.
Focus on your breathing.
On the outward breath, focus on the word 'calm' in your mind's eye, and say this internally.
Repeat this for five minutes.

Self-awareness relaxation – with script

In preparation for the finish of this relaxation, have a note pad and crayons or pens ready; when the relaxation has ended draw or write whatever images come in to your mind. You can discuss these with a like-minded friend afterwards to discover any meaning.

- Sit or lie in a comfortable position (see relaxation and meditation postures).
- Allow your body to relax and lengthen.
- Allow the muscles to soften.
- Focus your awareness on your breathing.
- Notice the depth and pace of your breathing.
- Allow your breathing to become slower, softer and deeper.
- Take your mind's awareness to your body.
- Notice any tightness or sensations in your body and give those areas your attention.
- Tell them you are aware and that you notice and acknowledge the feelings and sensations.
- Let the body be still and relaxed.
- Take your awareness to your mind.
- Notice the thoughts that enter your mind.
- Let the thoughts pass through, without holding on to any thought.

- Be the observer of your mind's activity.
- Focus deeper and inwards to yourself.
- See yourself as an object.
- What object do you notice?
- What colours are around you?
- What shape are you?
- What size are you?
- Are you still or moving?
- Notice all the details of the object.
- Notice any smells or sounds around the object.
- Take this object to one corner of your mind.
- Focus on how you experience your life.
- See your life experience as an object.
- What object do you notice?
- What colours are around this object?
- What shapes?
- What size is the object?
- Is the object still or moving?
- Notice all the details.
- Notice any smells or sounds around.
- Take this object to a different corner of your mind.
- Focus deeper.
- Allow your breathing to become slower and deeper.
- With every breath allow the body to relax further.
- Bring both the objects together into the foreground of your mind.
- Let them form a new image.
- Notice how the objects are positioned together in this new image.
- Notice their position and relationship to each other.
- Notice the colours, the sounds, smells, size and shapes.
- Observe the image.
- Focus fully on the image.
- Now bring your attention back into the room.
- Let your body slowly wake up and return to the awareness of the room.
- If you need to be still for a little while that is OK.

- You can wiggle your toes and fingers and open your eyes.
- When you are ready move steadily and take a paper and pens and draw the final picture you see... let it unfold.

Lifestyle habits

Diet and nutrition

The foods we eat will affect how much energy we have. They will also affect our health and well-being. It is worth remembering that there are no bad foods, just poor diets. It is therefore essential that we eat a balanced diet from the main food groups. These include: carbohydrates (pasta, potatoes, bread); fats (cheese, milk, butter); proteins (beans, pulses, meat); vitamins and minerals (vegetables and fruit); and water. We should also ensure that the quantity of food we consume is appropriate to meet our requirements.

Taking part in regular physical activity can make us more aware of the food we eat and more conscious of our diet. *The Complete Guide to Sports Nutrition* (A & C Black, 2003) provides the relevant information about this aspect of total fitness. Some general rules for improving our diet are:

- Eat less saturated fat. Too much will increase the risk of high cholesterol and increase furring of the artery walls.
- Eat less sugar. Too much will cause tooth decay and promote the risk of adult-onset (type II) diabetes. Too many refined foods will also imbalance blood sugar levels. They provide an initial pick-me-up and then energy levels drop.
- Eat less salt. Too much will potentially elevate blood pressure.
- Eat more complex carbohydrates. Too little will lower our energy levels.
- Eat sufficient fibre. Too little will potentially cause constipation and other bowel disorders.

- Eat a sufficient calorie intake. Too little will slow down our metabolism and make us feel lethargic, too much will make us put on weight and will be stored as body fat.
- Drink more water. Too little fluid will cause dehydration and potential heat stroke and place an unnecessary stress on the heart.
- Drink less coffee. Caffeine is a stimulant that actually triggers the stress response. After the initial pick-up, energy levels will drop.

After exercise the appetite is increased due to the energy and calories expended throughout the workout. The best time to replenish our glycogen stores (stored carbohydrate that we need for energy) is within two hours of activity. However, because many of us use exercise to assist with our weight management, it is worthwhile preparing a healthy and nutritious snack to eat after our activity. This will possibly reduce the temptation for us to purchase and consume a less nutritious snack. If we can plan our exercise programme, we can also plan our diet.

Alcohol

Alcohol can initially provide a relaxing effect and if used in moderation is acceptable. However, it can be easy to develop a habit of using alcohol to unwind. Excess alcohol can actually increase stress levels in the long term as they can contribute to a chemical imbalance in the body and disturb sleep patterns. Too much alcohol can also have other detrimental effects on our health and well-being. Persons who are concerned about their alcohol intake are advised to seek professional help from a specialist counsellor.

Smoking cessation

The negative consequences of cigarette smoking are well documented. Cigarettes can provide an initial effect of calming the body, but in the long term the build-up of toxins from cigarettes will actually raise stress levels by causing the heart rate to increase and creating a chemical imbalance. Smoking is addictive and quitting is not easy. Persons who wish to stop smoking are advised to contact a local smoking cessation group to receive advice and support to help them quit.

> *'Habit is habit, and not to be flung out of the window, but coaxed downstairs a step at a time.'*
>
> *Mark Twain*

Stress relief

Add some positive habits into your life and make exchanges for some of the less positive habits:

Drink herbal tea (peppermint or chamomile) instead of some caffeine drinks.

Smoke a herbal cigarette instead of the nicotine- and chemical-filled cigarettes.

Take a few deep breaths instead of having a cigarette (use the hand-to-mouth action if necessary or try a different movement pattern of your hand while you breathe).

Take a short walk before sitting down and having a glass of wine. After the walk you may find you don't need the alcohol.

Drink a glass of hot milk. Milk has a calming and nurturing effect.

Eat more fruit and vegetables as snacks throughout the day.

Drink more water.

NB: These ideas are only suggestions.

Desk mobility exercises

When we are at work, most of us will encounter some stress. It is useful to combat the physical symptoms of stress immediately as they arise. Persons who work in an office can perform some of the exercises listed below to combat the physical symptoms of stress while sitting at their desk. Time out to perform these exercises can also be used to replace other negative behaviours used to manage stress while at work, such as smoking or drinking coffee.

Ex 5.2	Shoulder lifts and rolls

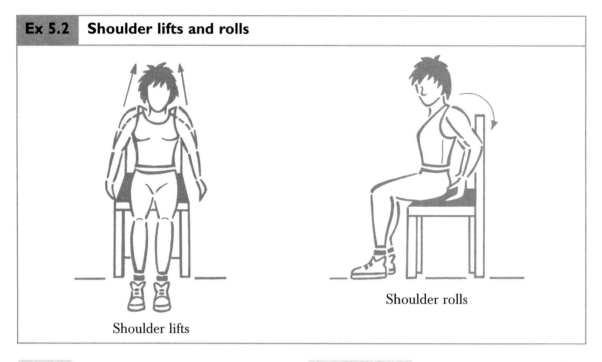

Shoulder rolls

Shoulder lifts

Purpose

These exercises mobilise the shoulder joint and can release tension around the neck and shoulder area.

Starting position and instructions

- Sit with the feet hip-width apart.
- Shoulder lifts – lift alternate shoulders towards the ears or both shoulders together.
- Shoulder rolls – roll alternate shoulders backwards or roll both shoulders together. These exercises can be performed for the desired number of repetitions.

Coaching points

1. Maintain an upright posture with the back straight and chest lifted.
2. Tighten the abdominal muscles.
3. Move the shoulders at a controlled speed and progressively aim to move through a larger range of motion.

Ex 5.3	Side bends (mobility)

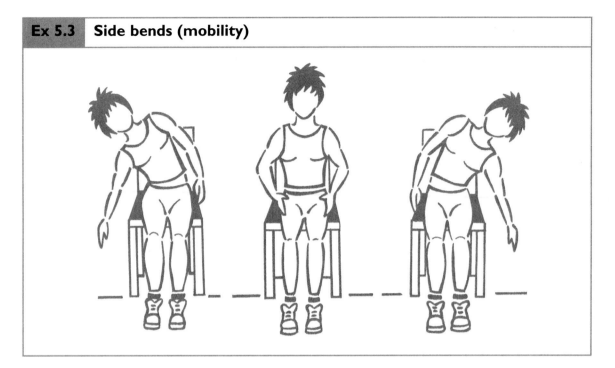

Purpose

This exercise will mobilise the thoracic vertebrae of the spine and release tension in the muscles around the trunk.

Starting position and instructions

- Sit with the feet hip-width apart and the body upright.
- Bend directly to the right side in a controlled manner.
- Return to the central position.
- Bend directly to the left side in a controlled manner.
- Return to the central position.
- Perform for the desired number of repetitions.

Coaching points

1. Bend only as far over as is comfortable.
2. Keep the hips facing forwards and avoid hollowing of the lower back by tightening the abdominal muscles.
3. Keep the movement controlled.
4. Keep the body lifted between the hips and the ribs.
5. Lift up before bending to the side.
6. Lean directly to the side and ensure the body does not roll forwards or backwards.
7. Visualise the body as being placed between two panes of glass.

Ex 5.4 Side twists

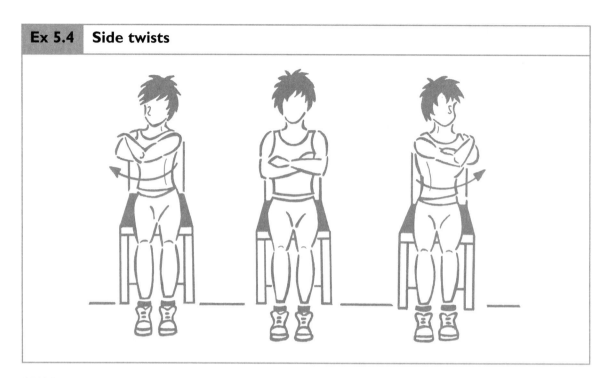

Purpose

This exercise will mobilise the thoracic vertebrae of the spine and release tension from the muscles around the trunk.

Starting position and instructions

- Sit with the feet hip-width apart.
- Hold the arms at shoulder level with the elbows slightly bent.
- Twist around to one side, back to centre and then again to the other side.

Coaching points

1. Keep the hips facing forwards.
2. Make sure the lower back does not twist.
3. Keep the abdominals pulled in.
4. Keep the chest lifted and the shoulders relaxed and down.
5. Keep a space between the shoulders and the ears and keep the neck long.

Ex 5.5	Heel and toe

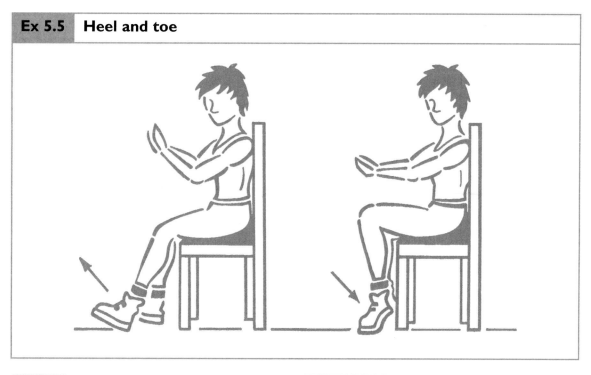

Purpose

This exercise mobilises the ankle joint and will release tension from the muscles of the lower leg.

Starting position and instructions

- Sit upright with the feet hip-width apart.
- Step one leg slightly forward and dig the heel to the floor.
- Then point the toe towards the floor, aiming to find the same spot the heel was on.
- Repeat for the desired number of repetitions and then perform on the other leg.

Coaching points

1. Keep the hips facing forwards and the back straight.
2. Keep the movement controlled
3. Keep the abdominals pulled in tightly.
4. Keep the shoulders relaxed and down and maintain a space between the shoulders and the ears.

| Ex 5.6 | **Back of thigh stretch** |

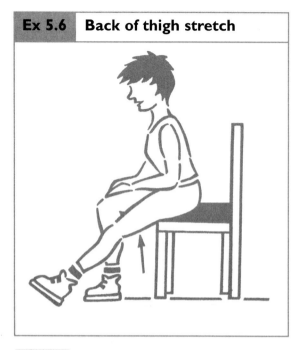

Purpose

This exercise lengthens, stretches and releases tension from the hamstring muscles at the back of the thigh, and also the buttock muscles, the gluteals.

Starting position and instructions

- Sit upright with feet hip-width apart, knees bent.
- Step one leg forward and extend the knee.
- Place the hands at the top of the thigh of the bent knee.
- Bend forward from the hip until a mild tension is felt at the back of the thigh on the straight leg.
- Repeat on the other leg.

Coaching points

1. Only bend forward to a point where a mild tension is felt at the back of the thigh.
2. Keep the knee of the straight leg fully extended, but not locked out.

3. Keep the hips square and pull the abdominals in to avoid hollowing the lower back.
4. Keep the spine long and the chest lifted.

| Ex 5.7 | **Calf stretch** |

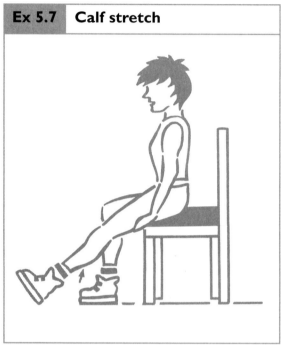

Purpose

This exercise lengthens, stretches and releases tension from the gastrocnemius and soleus muscles at the back of the lower leg.

Starting position and instructions

- Sit upright with the feet positioned at hip width apart, knees bent.
- Straighten one leg out to the front and flex the foot towards the knee
- Repeat on the other leg.

Coaching points

1. Keep the chest lifted and the abdominals pulled in.
2. Keep the knee unlocked.

| Ex 5.8 | Inner thigh stretch | Ex 5.9 | Side stretch |

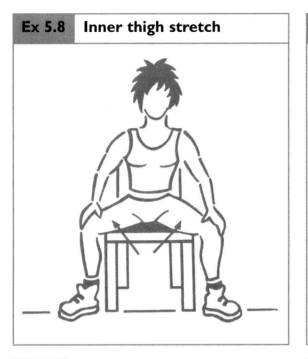

Purpose

This exercise lengthens, stretches and releases tension from the adductor muscles at the inside of the thigh.

Starting position and instructions

- Sit upright with the legs hip-width apart.
- Widen the legs as far as is comfortable
- Place the hands inside the knees and ease the knees outward slightly.

Coaching points

1. Step the legs further apart to increase the stretch of the inner thigh and groin.
2. Keep the hips facing forwards, the spine lengthened and the chest lifted.

Purpose

This exercise lengthens, stretches and releases tension from the muscles at the side of the trunk and side of the back, the obliques and latissimus dorsi.

Starting position and instructions

- Sit upright with the feet hip-width apart.
- Place the right hand on the side of the chair.
- Lift the left arm up and bend over slightly to the right side.

Coaching points

1. Emphasise lifting the body upwards rather than leaning too far over to the side.
2. Stretch only to a point of mild tension.
3. Keep a space between the shoulders and the ears and lengthen the neck.
4. When bending to the side, move the body in a straight line, not forwards or backwards.
5. Lift the ribcage upwards before bending to the side.

Ex 5.10	Back of the upper arm stretch

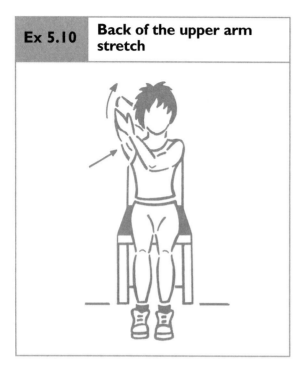

Ex 5.11	Chest stretch

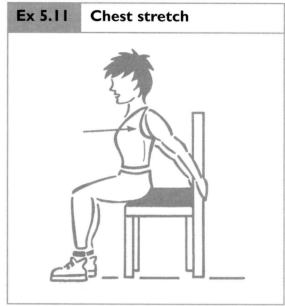

Purpose

This exercise lengthens, stretches and releases tension from the triceps muscles at the back of the upper arm.

Starting position and instructions

- Sit upright with the feet hip-width apart.
- Place one hand on the shoulder and gradually walk it down towards the centre of the back and use the other arm to ease the arm further back; hold still.

Coaching points

1. Keep the hips facing forwards and avoid hollowing of the lower back by pulling the abdominals in.
2. Stretch only to a point where a mild tension is felt at the back of the upper arm.

Purpose

This exercise lengthens, stretches and releases tension from the muscles of the chest, the pectorals.

Starting position and instructions

- Sit upright with the feet hip-width apart.
- Take the hands backwards and hold the back of the chair, lean forwards slightly until a mild tension is felt at the front of the chest.
- Alternatively, the hands can be placed on the buttocks or the hands can be clasped together behind the back, whichever is most comfortable.

Coaching points

1. Keep the elbows slightly bent.
2. Squeeze the shoulder blades together and lift the chest to increase the stretch.
3. Keep the hips facing forwards and avoid hollowing of the lower back by tightening the abdominal muscles.
4. Keep a space between the shoulders and ears and lengthen the neck.

Ex 5.12 | Middle back stretch

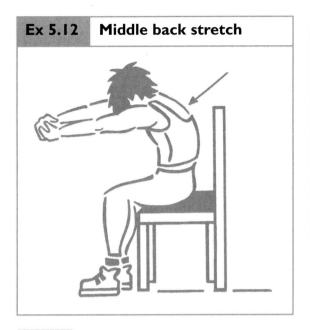

Purpose

This exercise stretches, lengthens and releases tension in the muscles in the middle of the back, the trapezius.

Starting position and instructions

- Sit upright with the feet hip-width-and-a-half apart.
- Take both arms forward in front of the body, just below shoulder height, and link the fingers.
- Round the shoulders over slightly to feel a mild tension in the middle of the upper back.

Coaching points

1. Keep the elbows slightly bent.
2. Keep the hips facing forwards and avoid hollowing of the lower back by tightening the abdominal muscles.
3. Round the shoulders over slightly but without leaning forwards at the hips.
4. Keep a space between the shoulders and the ears, lengthen the neck and make sure the shoulders do not hunch upwards.

EXERCISING AWAY STRESS

6

Physical activity

Why is physical activity important?

Physical activity plays a significant role in the promotion of good health. An active lifestyle can help to prevent many medical and mental health problems. For those of us who learn this lesson a little late, physical activity can, fortunately, also provide a major impact on alleviating some of the signs and symptoms of medical and mental health problems and will therefore improve our general well-being.

Modern lifestyles and the gadgets available to us (cars, washing machines, dish washers, elevators, escalators and so on) remove many naturally occurring opportunities for physical activity. Additionally, the increasingly fast pace of life and living seems to demand that much more needs to get done in less time. As a result of this, it would appear that physical activity and exercise become less of a priority.

Since most personal trainers will be fully aware of the general methods of promoting physical activity and exercise, the guidelines provided in this book will be comparatively few. Persons with the desire to further their knowledge in this area are guided to other texts in the *Complete Guide* series, listed at the front of this book. Table 6.1 provides a guide to the recommended levels of activity for persons who have been inactive; table 6.2 provides a list of possible activities for them to perform; and table 6.3 outlines the Borg Rate of Perceived Exertion scale for monitoring exercise intensity.

> ### Instant stress relief
>
> Stop what you are doing.
> Put on a track of music you like listening to and let your body dance freely to the music.

Table 6.1	Guidelines for increasing daily activity levels
Frequency	Work towards including activities in your daily routine on five days of the week
Intensity	Work at a level where you feel mildly breathless, warm but comfortable (use the adapted RPE intensity scale provided in table 6.3 and aim to work between levels 3 and 4)
Time	Work towards performing the chosen activities for a total of 30 minutes (this can initially be broken down into 3 x 10 minute slots of activity or 2 x 15 minute slots of activity), each day
Type	Any activity that fits well into your daily lifestyle! (Table 6.3 provides a list of activities) (NB: The list provided is not exhaustive! Moreover, it is just a start.)

Table 6.2	A list of possible activities	
Walking the dog	Cleaning house windows	Cleaning the car
Walking to and/or from the station (before and after work)	Doing housework with vigour	Walking to the shops
Walking up stairs or escalators at, or on the way to, work	Vacuuming the house	Cleaning the bathroom
Changing the beds	Scrubbing the floor	Walking to the park in your lunch hour
Taking the kids to the swing park and playing with them	Any physical games	Playing catch
Walking around the supermarket before starting to shop	Carrying a basket around the supermarket instead of using a shopping trolley	Walking to the pub
Walking upstairs at home more often	Playing a piece of music and dancing to it	Choose any activity before you sit down in the evening
Giving your partner a cuddle	Sweeping the kitchen floor	Marching on the spot to a piece of music

Table 6.3	The adapted Borg RPE (rate of perceived exertion) scale for monitoring exercise intensity		
Number:	Feels like:	Number:	Feels like:
0	Nothing	5	Getting harder
0.1	Very, very light	6	Hard
1	Very light	7	Harder
2	Light	8	Very hard
3	Moderate	9	Very, very hard
4	Somewhat hard	10	Maximum

Aim to work at a level between 3 and 4 when performing activities

Weekly activity log

A weekly activity log can be used to assist clients with managing time to programme physical activity. It can also act as a motivational tool to assist clients with monitoring and developing their activity level progress. Table 6.4 provides an outline of a weekly activity log used with one of my clients with other stress management techniques programmed.

Instant stress relief

Go for a short walk. It will definitely make you feel better.

Ideally, find a park or a space where there are lots of trees and where you can breathe in some fresh air. If you work in a built-up area, it is still good to find a space where there are lots of trees and flowers. Being close to natural things is a great way of helping us to appreciate the most valuable things in life, which are free!

Table 6.4	Weekly activity log for case study 1			
Day/Date	6am–10am	10am–2pm	2pm–6pm	6pm onwards
Monday	Walk to station Relaxation tape on train	Desk mobility exercises	Relaxation tape on way home	Walk from station Exercise class
Tuesday	Walk to station		Relaxation and breathing work 5 min	Walk from station Relaxing evening Creative drawing
Wednesday	Walk to station Relaxation tape on train	Desk mobility exercises		Walk from station Go walking with friend
Thursday	Walk to station Read self-help book on train			Walk from station Exercise class
Friday	Walk to station Read self-help book on train	Desk mobility exercises	Relaxation tape on way home	Walk from station
Saturday		Personal training gym session with steam room and jacuzzi afterwards Plan and complete weekly shop	Study time	Social
Sunday	Relax and read magazines	Clean house	Walk in park with friend	

NB: This diary can be used to plan other interventions. Part Four provides examples of how I have used it with other clients to assist their planning.

Exercising in water and swimming

As well as improving physical fitness, exercising in water and swimming provide additional benefits. Water is a naturally relaxing environment; a hot bath or jacuzzi can have a marvellous effect on relaxing the mind and the muscles. Exercising in water can provide similar relaxing and therapeutic effects. The reduced effects of the gravitational pull will automatically reduce some of the physical stress on the body. The increased effects of buoyancy will create flotation of the limbs, allowing the muscles to relax slightly. It will also support the weight of the body, decreasing the compression of the joints and allowing them to move more freely and with greater ease. The hydrostatic pressure exerted against the body will promote the circulation of a greater volume of blood and assist with removal of waste products that potentially may contribute to physical tension. In addition, the combined effects of hydrostatic pressure and the turbulence of the water against our bodies can provide a massaging effect. This will potentially decrease both physical and mental tension, promoting relaxation of the muscles and mind. There is also some evidence that immersion in water will reduce the activity of the sympathetic nervous system, which is most active during times of stress when we are preparing for fight or flight (Hall 1994).

However, while exercising in water and swimming can provide a stimulating and invigorating workout, which reduces tension and physical stress, it is worth noting that some participants, who are less confident in water, may not experience quite the same levels of relaxation as a confident participant! Further benefits, training considerations and programme designs for exercising in water can be found in the *Complete Guide to Exercise in Water* (2nd edition), A & C Black, 2004.

Running, jogging and walking

Running, jogging and walking are excellent methods for improving cardiovascular fitness. They are also very good ways of exercising away stress in the large muscles of the legs, which are likely to become activated for flight during times of stress. The benefits, training considerations and programme designs for each of these training methods is explored in other books in the *Complete Guide* series. Beginners to these types of activities are advised to join a club or group to ensure they receive appropriate advice about the frequency, intensity and duration of exercise appropriate to their needs.

Weight training

Weight training is an excellent way of improving muscular strength and endurance and can help to release tension built up in the upper body in response to the fight aspect of the stress mechanism. Working out in a gym is also a good way of meeting people and improving opportunities for socialisation, which can impact mental and emotional well-being. The benefits, training considerations and programme design for strength training are provided in the *Complete Guide to Strength Training* (3rd edition, A & C Black, 2005)

Group exercise

There are numerous types of group exercise classes that focus on improving different components of fitness. Table 6.5 lists a range of studio classes available and the primary fitness component improved. All sessions should include an adequate warm-up and cool-down and stretching activities should be included. Each type of session will have a good, albeit

Table 6.5	The range of group studio classes and the fitness component trained
Group studio training programme	*Component of fitness predominantly trained*
Studio cycling and studio rowing	Muscular endurance and cardiovascular fitness
Studio resistance	Muscular strength and endurance
Aerobic dance and step training to music	Cardiovascular fitness and muscular endurance
Body conditioning; legs, bums and tums	Muscular strength and endurance, some low-impact cardiovascular fitness
Circuit training	Muscular strength and endurance, cardiovascular fitness
Studio flexibility, Pilates and yoga	Flexibility, muscular strength and endurance, core muscle strength
Studio combat	Cardiovascular fitness, muscular strength and endurance

NB: The names of different sessions will vary between different clubs. Some branded group exercise sessions can be led only by instructors who have attended specific training.

different, effect on reducing stress depending on the component they focus on training.

The greatest benefit of any group exercise session is that it provides a social environment. Social support systems are essential for human beings to thrive. Group exercise appears to be particularly effective for improving our social fitness. This may be due to the fact that it is a group activity that naturally encourages networking and friendships to blossom among class members. The social activities that occur after the sessions are all due to relationships being developed between class members. The sessions use partner work, themed workouts and group activities specifically to lighten the atmosphere and encourage interaction among class members. Group exercise enhances communication and promotes the development of friendships between a wide range of participants.

The benefits, training considerations and specific programme design for circuit training, exercise to music and core stability are provided in other books in the *Complete Guide* series.

Stress relief tip

Join an exercise class at your local leisure centre. Try a few different sessions until you find one you really enjoy.

Pilates

Pilates is a fabulous way of improving posture and alignment. It emphasises slow and controlled movement that focuses the mind and breathing, and works on the deeper core muscles of the abdominals, shoulder girdle, spine and middle back that help to keep the body aligned and stable throughout all other movements. The Pilates method works with eight principles in mind:

- balance
- breathing
- stamina
- co-ordination
- concentration
- flowing movement
- alignment
- centring.

The technique is named after its creator, Joseph Pilates, who, after experimenting with a variety of different exercise disciplines such as yoga, gymnastics, weight training, dance and self defence, developed his own programme of exercises to overcome his own health problems (asthma, rickets, and rheumatic fever). The technique has become highly regarded around the world and increasingly popular in the last decade. Some introductory exercises to strengthen the core muscles that are based on the Pilates method are provided on the following pages. A list of training organisations who specialise in Pilates teacher training are provided at the back of this book.

> 'Pilates is the single most effective exercise technique I have ever known'
>
> Stefanie Powers (actress)

Exercise guidelines

Before starting an exercise programme, it is wise to speak with your GP if you have any specific concerns about your medical health that may affect participation.

Always inform your personal trainer or instructor of any changes to your medical health.

Always start your exercise programme gently and build up the programme gradually.

Make sure you warm up and cool down thoroughly.

Ex 6.1	Pelvic tilt

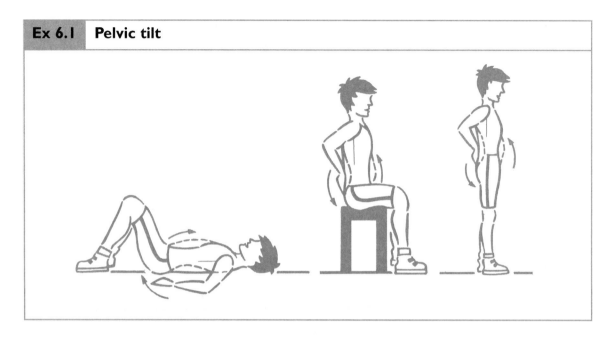

Purpose

To find the neutral pelvic position. This movement needs to be maintained during abdominal work and other exercises to ensure the lumbar spine does not move excessively.

Starting position and instructions

Lying:
- Lie on your back with knees bent.
- Keep your feet hip-width apart.
- Relax your shoulders and neck.
- Lengthen the spine.

Seated:
- Sit on the sitting bones (you can feel these in the middle of each buttock cheek).
- Sit upright and tall.

Standing:
- Keep feet hip-width apart.
- Lengthen spine, stand upright.

Teaching points

1. Tighten the abdominals and buttocks to tilt the pelvis backwards (the pubic bone will press up and the lower back will press to the floor or the lower spine will flatten).
2. Tighten the hips and back to tilt the pelvis forwards (the pubic bone lowers and the small of the back hollows).
3. Repeat this a few times.
4. Find a midway point between these two movements and hold the pelvis still. This is the neutral pelvic position.
5. Control the movement.
6. Breathe comfortably throughout.

Progressions/adaptations/variations

As a variation, perform this exercise seated or standing (keep your spine upright and make sure the movement is isolated and the rest of the body remains still).

Ex 6.2 Abdominal hollowing

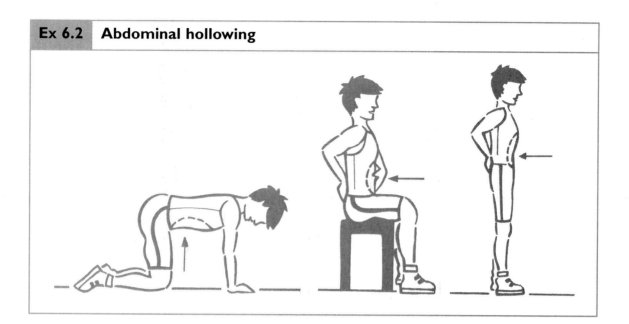

Purpose

To work the muscles that help to control movement and stabilise the spine.

Starting position

Kneeling:

- Place your hands and knees on the floor, shoulder-width apart.
- Find a neutral pelvic position.
- Tighten the tummy muscles and pull the tummy button towards the spine.

Seated:

- Sit upright and lengthen the spine.
- Keep the feet hip-width apart.
- Find a neutral pelvic position.

Standing:

- Keep the feet hip-width apart, with your weight distributed evenly between the heel, big toe and little toe.
- Find a neutral pelvic position.

Teaching points

1. Breathe normally throughout or breathe out when pulling the tummy in.
2. Keep the pelvis, spine and shoulders still.
3. Make sure the back doesn't flatten.
4. Keep the shoulders relaxed and the neck lengthened.
5. Keep elbows unlocked.

Progressions/adaptations/variations

- The movement of the tummy will be small at first; as the muscles get stronger, progress by pulling the tummy in further.
- Perform in a seated position on a chair and progress to a stability ball.
- Perform standing.

Rest

Child pose (if kneeling).

Ex 6.3 | Heel slide

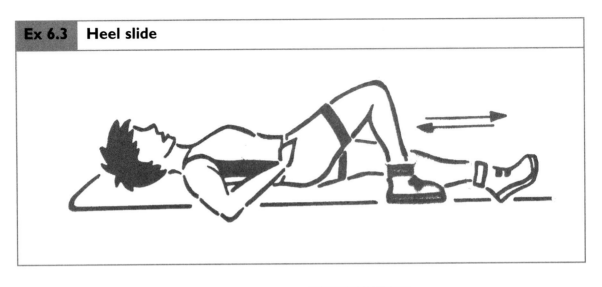

Purpose

To strengthen the muscles that hold the pelvis still.

Starting position and instructions

- Lie on your back, feet hip-width apart.
- Find a neutral pelvis position.
- Place your hands on the pelvic bones (to monitor movement of pelvis).
- Your legs need to be able to slide along the floor, so perform the exercise without shoes – socks slide more easily.
- The shoulders need to be relaxed and the spine lengthened.

Teaching points

1. Pull your tummy in tight without moving the pelvis (abdominal hollowing).
2. Breathe normally throughout the exercise.
3. Slide your leg along the floor until you feel the pelvis begin to tilt. At this point pause and slide your leg back to its original position.
4. Repeat with the other leg.
5. Make sure your legs do not lift off the floor.
6. Alternative breathing: on the outward breath, pull the tummy tight and commence leg sliding action. Breathe in, and breathe out, contracting the abdominals to slide the leg back to the start position.

Ex 6.4 Reciprocal reach

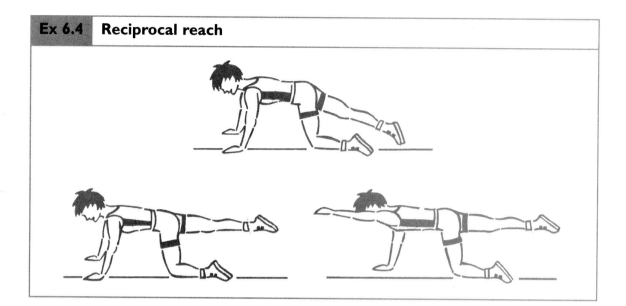

Level 1 – Leg only to rear
Level 2 – Leg only to hip height
Level 3 – Leg and arm to hip height

Purpose

To strengthen the muscles that maintain the neutral pelvic position and stabilise the spine. To develop balance and control.

Starting position and instructions

- Place your hands and knees on the floor directly underneath the hips and shoulders.
- Find neutral pelvis position.
- Breathe in and lengthen the spine.

Level 1
- Breathe out, and hollow and tighten the abdominals, sliding your right leg backwards.
- Breathe in and return the leg to the centre.
- Repeat with the other leg.

Level 2
- Breathe out, hollow and tighten the abdominals, slide your right leg backwards and raise it to hip height.

- Breathe in and return the leg to the centre.
- Repeat with the other leg.

Level 3
- Breathe out, hollow and tighten the abdominals, slide and raise your right leg to hip height and at the same time extend your left arm forwards to shoulder height.
- Breathe in and return the leg and arm to the centre.

Teaching points

1. Maintain a neutral pelvis throughout.
2. Keep the abdominals tight throughout.
3. Keep the spine lengthened.
4. Keep the weight evenly distributed through both hands.
5. Make sure the back doesn't dip.
6. Make sure the pelvis doesn't tilt to one side.

Level 3
7. Keep the shoulder blades square and the neck and spine lengthened.

Rest

Child pose.

Yoga

Yoga is an excellent way of improving flexibility, balance and strength. Exercise technique, posture, breathing and mental awareness of the body are all emphasised in this type of exercise programme. Yoga is based on deeper spiritual awareness and philosophy and in some sessions this will also be emphasised. There are various forms of yoga; some are more calming and some are more dynamic. Individuals are advised to choose the type of session that meets their own needs and fitness. A list of web sites is provided at the end of this book.

Ex 6.5	Mountain pose

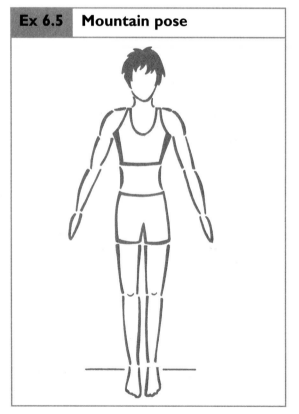

Purpose

A starting position for all other standing postures. Can be used as a rest to centre the body between postures.

Starting position and instructions

- Stand with your feet together or parallel.
- Lengthen your spine and relax your shoulders.
- Find neutral pelvis position with the abdominals hollowed.
- Distribute your weight evenly between your big toes, little toes and heel-bones.
- Look straight ahead with your neck lengthened.
- Hold your arms slightly away from the sides of your body, lengthening through the fingers.
- Breathe naturally.

Ex 6.6 Arm raise and prayer pose

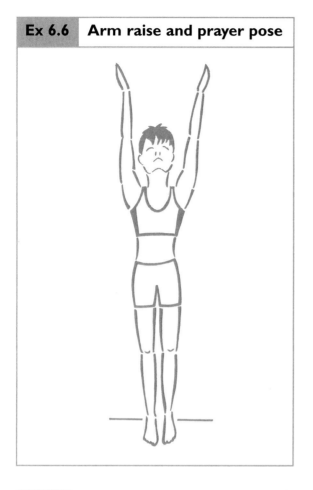

Purpose

To raise awareness of breathing while synchronising movement of the upper body.

Starting position and instructions

- Stand in mountain pose.
- Breathe in, raise your arms out to the sides of your body and, reaching above your head, look up slightly.
- Breathe out, placing your palms together in a prayer position and lower your arms to chest level, looking straight ahead.
- Breathe in, raise your arms up into a prayer position above your head, looking up slightly.
- Breathe out and lower your arms back down to the sides of your body, looking straight ahead.
- Rest and repeat.

Teaching points

1. Maintain a neutral pelvis position.
2. Keep the spine lengthened.
3. Keep the shoulders relaxed and neck long.

Rest

Mountain pose.

Ex 6.7 Chair pose

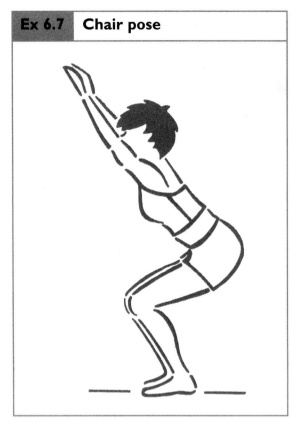

Purpose

A strong, dynamic movement that will raise the heart rate, increase circulation and warm the body when performed repeatedly and rhythmically. It will also strengthen the muscles of the thighs and buttocks (quadriceps, hamstrings and gluteals).

Starting position and instructions

- Start in mountain pose, with your feet parallel and hip-width apart.
- Spread your weight evenly between the feet.
- Breathe in and lengthen the body.
- Breathe out and simultaneously bend your knees to 90 degrees and raise your arms in front of your body until they are close to your ears. Hands should touch lightly in prayer position.
- Hold for as long as is comfortable, breathing naturally.
- Lift out of the position on an outward breath (exhalation).
- Rest and repeat.

Teaching points

1. Keep the abdomen hollowed.
2. Look forwards and slightly up when arms are raised.
3. Maintain the length of the spine.
4. Keep your neck long and your shoulders relaxed.
5. Make sure the breath is not held.
6. Keep both feet firmly on the floor, with your weight spread evenly.

Adaptations

- Bend to a lesser angle that can be achieved comfortably.
- Raise the arms to a lower height.

Rest

Mountain pose.

Ex 6.8 Crane pose

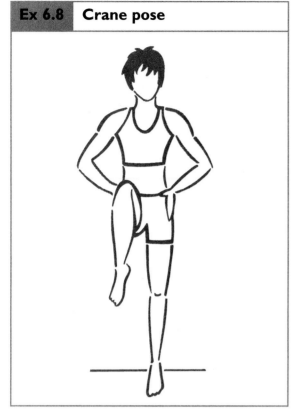

Purpose

To develop balance and stability. It is a starting point before attempting to perform other, more advanced standing postures.

Starting position and instructions

- Stand with your feet parallel and ankles as close together as possible; keep your arms at the sides of your body.
- Body weight should be distributed evenly between the big toe, little toe and heels of both feet.
- The arches of the feet should be lifted to prevent ankles rolling.
- Tighten your thigh muscles, drawing the kneecaps upwards.
- Take your body weight on one leg and place your hands on the pelvic bones.
- Raise your other leg so that the knee is slightly higher than the hip and the foot is in line under the hip.
- Lower your leg and repeat on the other side.

Teaching points

1. Maintain a neutral pelvis position.
2. Keep your spine lengthened and abdominals tight (abdominal hollowing).
3. Keep your chest open and neck lengthened.
4. Breathe comfortably throughout.

Adaptation

Lift leg to hip height or lower if flexibility is limited.

Rest

Mountain pose.

Ex 6.9 | Tree pose

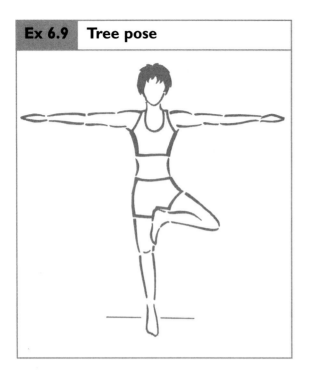

Purpose

To develop balance and stability and open up the hip joint. Helps to focus the mind.

Starting position and instructions

- Stand with your feet parallel and ankles as close together as possible.
- Body weight should be distributed evenly between your big toe, little toe and heels of both feet.
- The arches of the feet should be lifted to prevent ankles rolling.
- Tighten the thigh muscles, drawing the kneecaps upwards.
- Take your body weight on one leg.
- Raise your other leg and take hold of the ankle.
- Place the foot of the raised leg on the inside thigh of the supporting leg.
- Take your arms to the sides of your body, level with your shoulders and parallel to the floor.
- Turn the knee outwards on the bent leg to open up the hip.
- Lower your leg and repeat on the other side.

Teaching points

1. Maintain a neutral pelvis position.
2. Keep your spine lengthened and your abdominals tight (abdominal hollowing).
3. Keep your chest open and your neck lengthened.
4. Breathe comfortably throughout.

Adaptation

Place your leg slightly lower, either above or below the knee, to accommodate limited flexibility.

Rest

Mountain pose.

Ex 6.10 Staff pose

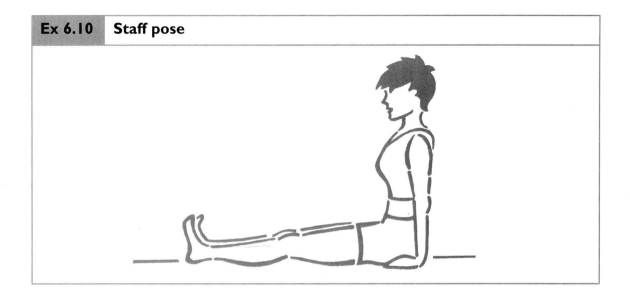

Purpose

Basic sitting position that prepares for other seated postures. Challenging when performed correctly and held for a few breaths.

Starting position and instructions

- Sit upright, fully onto the sitting bones with your legs out straight.
- Place your hands on the floor beside your hips.
- Spread your toes, pressing the balls of the feet lightly away from your body.

Teaching points

1. Lengthen and hollow the abdominals.
2. Maintain a neutral pelvis position by keeping the core muscles strong, yet soft.
3. Keep your shoulders relaxed and spine lengthened.
4. Keep your knees unlocked.

Adaptation

Sit with the back against a wall to assist with supporting the spine.

Rest

Bend your knees and let your body rest forwards over your thighs.

Ex 6.11 Forward stretch

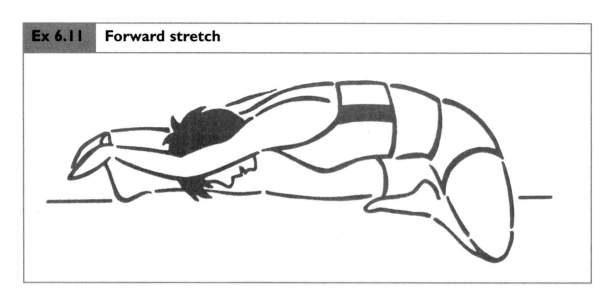

Purpose

Relaxes and lengthens the spine and lengthens the muscles at the back of the thigh (hamstrings).

Starting positions and instructions

- Sit in staff pose (see page 97).
- Bend one leg and place the sole of your foot on the inside of the thigh as close to the pubic bone as comfortable.
- Breathe in, opening the chest and lengthening the spine.
- Breathe out and bend forwards at the hip, reaching your hands forwards to take hold of the foot.
- Breathe in, lengthening your spine and neck, and lifting the chin slightly.
- Breathe out, bend your arms and lengthen forwards further into the stretch.
- Breathe in, lengthening your spine and easing the crown of your head forwards.
- Hold the position for as long as is comfortable, breathing naturally.
- Breathe in to lengthen out of the stretch and back into staff pose.
- Rest, then repeat with the other leg.

Teaching points

1. Keep your spine lengthened and shoulders relaxed.
2. Lengthen and hollow the abdomen.
3. Keep your chest wide and relaxed.

Adaptation

Place one leg out to the side of the body at 90 degrees. Reach towards the toes, but place hands in a position that is comfortable.

Rest

Staff pose.

Ex 6.12   Easy boat pose

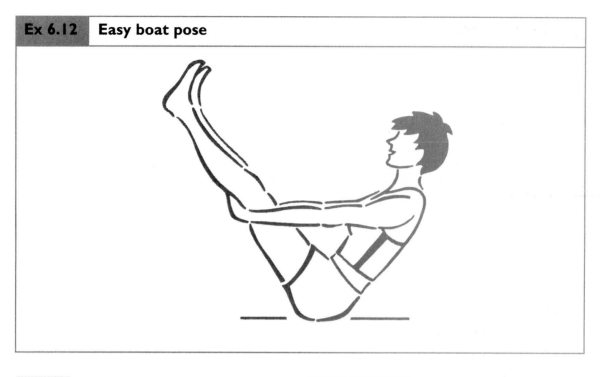

Purpose

To develop balance and strengthen the legs and core stabilisers.

Starting position and instructions

- Sit on the floor with your legs bent and spine lengthened.
- Breathe in, taking your weight backwards onto your buttocks; take your feet off the floor and wrap your hands around the back of your thighs.
- Breathe out and extend your knees.
- Breathe in and bend your knees again.
- Breathe out and place your feet on the floor.

Teaching points

1. Maintain a neutral pelvis.
2. Keep your spine lengthened, shoulders relaxed and ribcage open.
3. Keep the abdominals tightened and hollow.

Progressions and adaptations

- To make the exercise easier, keep your knees bent at 90 degrees.
- To make the exercise harder, lengthen your arms to the sides of your legs.

Rest

Staff pose or rest for staff pose.

Ex 6.13	**Open pose**

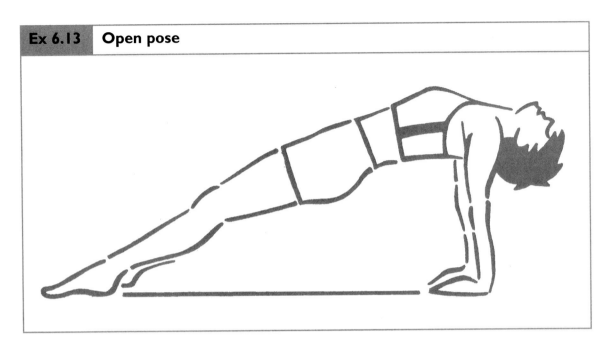

Purpose

To lengthen the muscles of the chest (pectorals) and the forearms.

Starting position and instructions

- Sit upright in staff pose.
- Breathe in and lean back, sliding your hands backwards on the floor behind you. Keep your fingers facing forwards.
- Breathe out and straighten your arms, pressing your palms down.
- Breathe in and lift and open the chest, hollowing the back slightly.
- Hold for as long as is comfortable, breathing naturally.
- Breathe out to return to staff pose.
- Rest and repeat.

Teaching points

1. Keep your shoulders relaxed and spine lengthened.
2. Keep your abdominals hollowed.

Progressions and adaptations

- Bend your knees to adapt the pose.
- To progress the pose, keep your legs bent, lift your buttocks off the floor and press your hips upwards, maintaining a neutral pelvis position.
- To progress further, with straight legs, raise your buttocks off the floor so the whole body weight is supported between your hands and feet. Keep your body straight.

Rest

Staff pose or rest for staff pose.

Ex 6.14   Cat pose

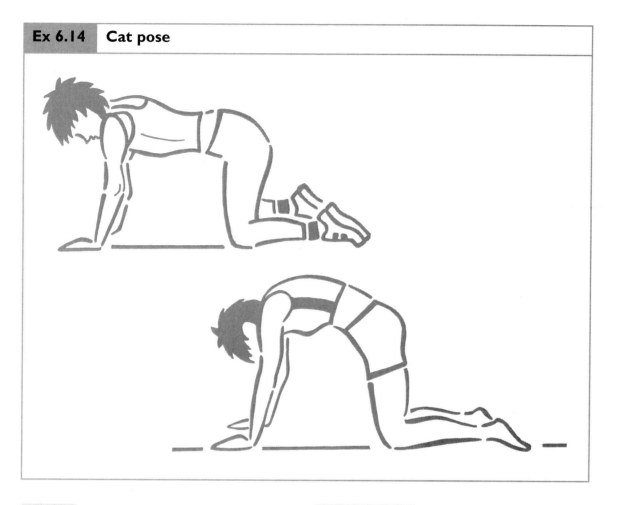

Purpose

To focus awareness on synchronisation of breathing while moving the spine. Increases mobility of the spine.

Starting position and instructions

- Position yourself on your hands and knees.
- Keep your hands underneath your shoulders.
- Keep your knees underneath your hips.
- Breathe in and hollow the spine slightly, tilting the tailbone in the air.
- Breathe out, tighten the abdominals and tuck the tailbone underneath, rounding the spine.
- Repeat.

Teaching points

1. Keep your neck and shoulders relaxed and lengthened.
2. Keep your weight spread evenly between your hands and knees.
3. Keep the movement slow and controlled.
4. Be aware of moving only within a comfortable range of motion within the limitations of your own body.

Rest

Child pose.

Ex 6.15 | Cat and dog pose

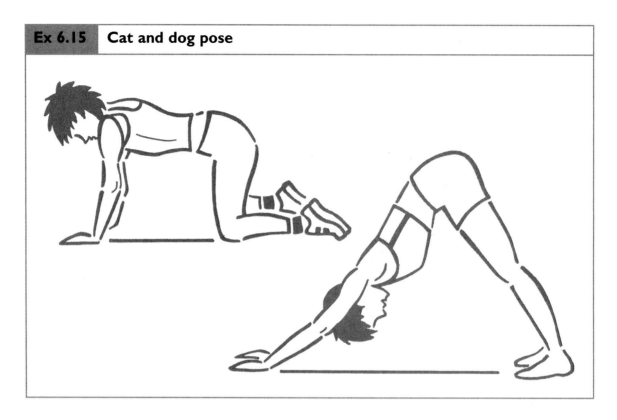

Purpose

To focus awareness on breathing. To lengthen the muscles at the back of the legs and buttocks and lower back. To strengthen the upper body.

Starting position and instructions

- Position yourself on your hands and knees.
- Keep your hands underneath your shoulders, weight distributed evenly between fingers, thumbs and balls of the hands.
- Keep your knees underneath your hips.
- Place the toes and balls of the feet on the floor with the heels up.
- Breathe in and hollow the spine slightly, tilting the tailbone in the air (cat pose).
- Breathe out, tighten the abdominals, and straighten your legs with the sitting bones pointing towards the ceiling (dog pose).
- Repeat.

Teaching points

1. Keep your neck, shoulders and head relaxed and lengthened.
2. Keep the weight spread evenly between your hands and knees/hands and feet.
3. Keep the movement slow and controlled.
4. Be aware of moving only within a comfortable range of motion within the limitations of your own body.
5. Keep your spine relaxed and lengthened.

Adaptation

Keep your knees slightly bent during the dog pose to reduce the stretch on the muscles at the back of the leg.

Rest

Child pose.

Ex 6.16 | **Child pose**

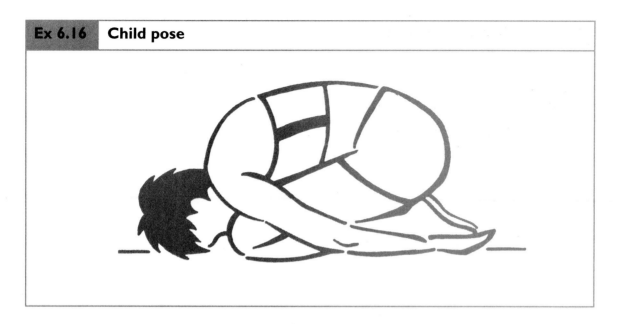

Purpose

To provide a restful position for the whole body. Can be used as a rest/relaxation between cat and dog pose or any other postures and exercises where the upper and lower body are used simultaneously and are bearing the body weight.

Starting position and instructions

- Start on your hands and knees.
- Slide your buttocks back to rest on your heels with your chest resting on your thighs.
- Slide your hands down to the sides of your body.
- Hold for as long as is comfortable.

Teaching points

1. Breathe comfortably throughout.
2. Relax your shoulders and neck.
3. Keep your spine lengthened.
4. Tighten and hollow the abdomen.

Adaptations

- Form two fists with your hands and place one on top of the other underneath your forehead to support the head and neck.
- Alternatively, lengthen your arms in front of your body.
- Keep the buttocks slightly away from the heels if flexibility of the spine is limited.

WORKING WITH CLIENTS WITH STRESS

This section of the book describes the trans-theoretical model for changing behaviour and identifies the strategies that can be used to promote positive movement through all stages of the change process.

It also identifies some of the skills and qualities that will enable personal trainers and fitness instructors to help clients with managing stress.

RAISING AWARENESS AND MAKING CHANGES

7

How can we raise awareness and assist change?

Prochaska and Diclemente (1984; in Feltham and Horton 2000) name ten common processes that people involved in a change and growth process move through. Some of the strategies that can be used are listed under each of these processes. (Feltham and Horton 2000: 400).

Consciousness-raising

Gathering information about oneself and the problem(s) to increase awareness. For example:

- keeping a stress diary
- writing a hassle list
- keeping a food diary to identify when one is triggered to eat certain foods
- keeping a smoking diary to identify when one is triggered to have a cigarette.

Self-liberation

Believing in the possibility of change and making the choice to commit to take action. For example:

- using the decisional balance sheet to assist making the decision to take back personal power and control
- finding the inner determination to commit to working with and handling the problem
- using positive self-talk to maintain the self-belief.

Social liberation

Raising awareness of the increasing opportunity for alternative behaviours in society. For example:

- stress management programmes
- assertiveness training
- GP referral exercise schemes
- diet and exercise clubs
- smoking cessation programmes.

Counter-conditioning

Introducing alternative behaviour to the specific problem behaviour. For example:

- taking a few deep breaths instead of having a cigarette
- going for a short walk before sitting down for the evening
- taking five minutes to sit and meditate before starting and finishing the day to increase positive thinking.

Stimulus control

Raising awareness of the stimuli that promote the problem behaviour and avoiding or resisting these stimuli. For example:

- keeping a diary to recognise what triggers specific behaviour and identifying personal strategies to avoid or resist the situation
- placing cigarettes in the boot of the car to avoid the impulse to smoke in traffic
- listening to a positive thinking tape while in the car to occupy the mind and focus on positive thoughts, and therefore avoid negative thinking patterns that cause stress and create other problem behaviour stimulus.

Self re-evaluation

Evaluating how one thinks and feels about oneself in relation to the problem behaviour. For example:

- speaking to a therapist or counsellor regarding stress and depression
- keeping a journal to recognise how one thinks about oneself in relation to the behaviour, for example 'When I get angry at my family I feel guilty and remorseful and then berate myself some more and I end up feeling really bad.' 'When I eat a whole box of biscuits I feel angry at myself for letting myself down and being weak-willed.'

Environmental re-evaluation

Recognising how the problem behaviour affects the broader physical community and environment. For example:

- recognising that smoking contributes to polluting the atmosphere
- recognising how one's bad moods, negative thinking and unassertive behaviours impact others, which may in turn affect their behaviour.

Contingency/reinforcement management

Being rewarded for making changes to behaviour either by oneself or others. For example:

- saving money spent from not smoking and treating oneself to a day at a health spa
- buying a new outfit for sticking to an exercise and/or relaxation programme.

Dramatic relief

Experiencing and expressing feelings that may be linked with the problem behaviour and identifying possible solutions to manage these. For example:

- working with a counsellor or support worker to discuss feelings
- working with a personal trainer to identify exercise and other activities to help manage stress levels
- writing a journal
- writing or drawing pictures to express feelings.

Helping relationships

Being able to trust and speak openly about problems with people who care. For example:

- speaking to a therapist or to close friends and family about the problems one is experiencing and would like to manage more effectively
- speaking to a personal trainer to find solutions to assist with managing stress through exercise.

The trans-theoretical model of change

This is one model used for behaviour change. It provides a number of stages that relate to where an individual may be positioned in relation to the change process. Identifying the position of an individual in the cycle of change can help to identify appropriate strategies to assist with helping the individual to change. Figure 7.1 provides a diagram of the trans-theoretical model of change.

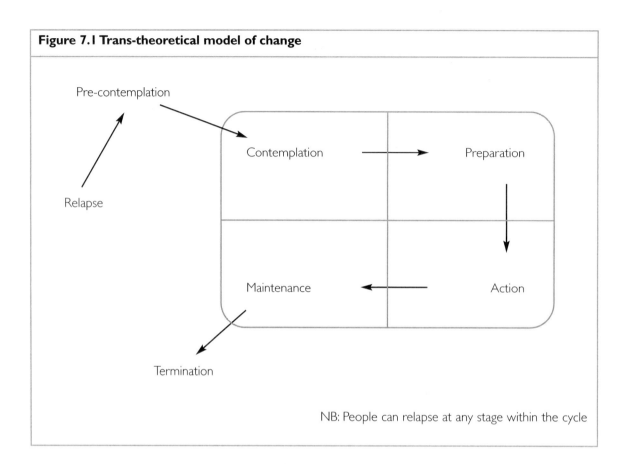

Figure 7.1 Trans-theoretical model of change

NB: People can relapse at any stage within the cycle

Stages of change and interventions

Pre-contemplation

At this stage of the change cycle individuals are not aware they have a problem and are not thinking about making any changes. There may be resistance to the change process due to feelings of powerlessness or helplessness or possibly because of a fear of failure.

At this stage the personal trainer can provide information that may assist the person to move closer towards contemplating making a change. They can give information in the form of handouts or leaflets that can help to raise the client's awareness of the risks associated with continuing his or her existing behaviour. They can also use sensitive motivational interviewing techniques in a supportive and non-judgemental environment, which can help clients explore their resistance and any fears they may hold in relation to making a change of behaviour. Validating how the client feels is important at this stage. Whatever a person feels is real for them, and feelings will continuously provide a barrier to change if their realness is not acknowledged.

The client's body language and non-verbal language can often provide an indication of defences and barriers that she or he is maintaining. The personal trainer can use open questioning techniques to enquire about these signs that the client is providing, if it feels appropriate to do so. An example is given in table 7.1.

Table 7.1	Example of pre-contemplation dialogue
	Pre-contemplation dialogue
Client:	My partner gave me this personal training session as a Christmas present. I don't really like training, I don't have time, but my partner thinks I am too stressed at work.
Trainer:	So you don't really like training or have time for it, but you are here because your partner thinks you are stressed and gave you this for Christmas?
Client:	That's right. She says I should start exercising before or after work but I don't have enough time and I am too tired then.
Trainer:	Too tired?
Client:	Yes. I work really long hours and have a really high-pressured work schedule.
Trainer:	High pressure?
Client:	Yes. I have deadlines to meet and they are a priority.
Trainer:	Your work deadlines are very important to you?
Client:	Yes they are. If I don't meet them, then I'm out of a job and we could lose the home etc...
Trainer:	How does that feel?
Client:	Well, it puts me under a lot of stress.
Trainer:	Stress?
Client:	Yes, sometimes it feels like I'll explode, but I have to get on with it.
Trainer:	Having to get on with it sounds really stressful and you use the word 'explode', that's a very powerful word.
Client:	Is it? It just means I feel like going aaaaarghh!!!!!!! sometimes.
Trainer:	Maybe you could go aaaaargghh!!! sometimes?
Client:	I don't think so, people would think I was crazy!
Trainer:	OK. How about if we use this session to explore some ways you could manage the aaarghhh feeling and look at ways of managing stress while you are at work? I can give you some ideas on ways to increase your activity without having to come to the gym when you are tired. I can also show you some relaxation techniques and give you some written information. How does that sound?
Client:	That sounds reasonable.

Contemplation

At this stage of the change process the individual is aware that a problem exists and is seriously considering making changes. He or she may experience internal conflicts regarding the advantages and disadvantages of making changes and may become stuck at this stage and move no further unless specific interventions are applied.

The personal trainer can help the client to explore the advantages and disadvantages of both changing and not changing and also explore the risk and harm caused by their existing behaviour. This can be done using the decisional balance sheet outlined in table 7.2.

The trainer can also explore the personal conflicts that the client may be experiencing. It may be that the client is fearful about making the changes and feels she or he will not be able to succeed. These issues need to be dealt with

sensitively and empathically as they are very real to the client's experience.

The choice to make changes lies with the client. If he or she is contemplating making a change it is essential to promote the benefits of that change, build commitment and confidence and reinforce the possibility that it can be done, that there is a way, and that the internal conflict can be managed and the desired changes made.

It is also worthwhile if the trainer encourages the client to use a diary to explore her or his behaviour. By keeping a diary the client will become more aware of things that may prevent changes being made. For example, 'I didn't go to the gym because I felt too tired.' It can also identify patterns of behaviour that are out of the client's awareness. For example, discovering that when they feel stressed they have another cup of coffee, which can actually increase stress levels. Keeping a diary will help to identify

Table 7.2	Decisional balance sheet	
	Advantages	Disadvantages
Change	1. 2. 3. 4. 5.	1. 2. 3. 4. 5.
No change	1. 2. 3. 4. 5.	1. 2. 3. 4. 5.

where simple strategies can be used to replace the existing behaviour, if the client wants to make these changes.

The diary can also raise awareness of the client's behaviour and provide a greater insight into ways that he or she could make changes that are comparatively simple. The trainer can point out these simpler ways and identify how much easier they would be to make. For example, a client who eats more junk food when she is stressed can be reminded that she could eat other, more nutritious foods, which would also help with her other goal of losing weight.

Preparation

At this stage of the change process the individual is ready to change and may have already made some small changes. They may have started a yoga class to help release stress or reduced their coffee intake during the day. However, they are still not fully committed to the change process as yet.

The personal trainer can help at this stage by exploring a variety of options to bring about the desired changes and can speak with the client to strengthen his or her commitment and build confidence towards making small changes. The trainer can help the client to make some goals

Table 7.3	Example of contemplation dialogue
	Contemplation dialogue
Client:	I feel really stressed and I would like to find some ways to make myself feel better.
Trainer:	It sounds like you are ready to make some positive changes for yourself to make you feel better.
Client:	Yes, I am... I'm just a little worried that I will start something and then give up because I don't have time and cannot motivate myself.
Trainer:	How about we look at a few possible strategies you can use and you can decide which ones may fit with your schedule? We can also look at ways you can get some extra motivation to help you on your way.
Client:	I just need to sort myself out, once this month is over I may be ready to do something.
Trainer:	That's great, maybe we can find some little ways you can start getting ready to make some changes now? One step at a time, rather than trying to do lots at once?
Client:	I guess we could, but I don't want to say I'm going to do something and then not do it because that will make me feel worse.
Trainer:	Absolutely. That's why it is important that we find things you feel comfortable to manage. It could be something really simple like saying some positive things to yourself.
Client:	Well, I guess that doesn't require too much effort at this stage!
Trainer:	It's one way of getting started. We can look at others. It is about finding what will work best for you.

Table 7.4	Example of preparation stage dialogue
	Preparation dialogue
Trainer:	How are you doing?
Client:	Well, I've attended my yoga class this week and I've also had my hair done, and I'm here today. Work is still the same. I couldn't come last week because as I was getting ready to leave my boss asked me to do something.
Trainer:	Sounds like you've made some positive steps towards finding time for yourself this week. Have you considered attending an assertiveness training course? This may help you to say no when its time to leave work.
Client:	No, I hadn't thought of that.
Trainer:	I think they run these at the local adult education centre, I will give you the number.
Client:	OK, that would be great.

(using the SMART method described in chapter 4) and establish an action plan for achieving these goals. See table 7.4 for a sample preparation stage dialogue.

Action

At this stage of the change process the individual is making changes and has committed some time and energy to the change process. She or he may have made the changes for just one day or up to six months.

The personal trainer can help at this stage by focusing on the client's successes and positively affirming progress. This positive reinforcement helps to maintain motivation and can build self-efficacy and help the client to stay committed. The trainer can also guide the client towards using positive affirmations or self-help strategies (suggested throughout this book) that will help him or her maintain motivation.

The trainer can also explore external stimuli that may trigger the behaviour and look at ways of avoiding or managing these stimuli (stimulus control). For example, smokers may wish to avoid going to the bar after work where they will be tempted to have a cigarette. An alternative behaviour could be proposed, such as attending an exercise session or any other activity that will distract from the stimulus.

The trainer could suggest that the client has a massage or another personal reward for maintaining a change of behaviour. They can also explore the client's feelings concerning the change and encourage the client to look at the positive impact of their new behaviour. For example, a client who is new to exercise could be encouraged to look at how he feels better after their exercise session, even though he feels tired before he attends. This exploration of both the positive and negative aspects of the change can provide reinforcement that helps to maintain and manage the change of behaviour.

It can also be useful to explore a range of alternative behaviours and other coping strategies. For example, a client who drinks a cup of coffee when stressed could explore the option of drinking other beverages that will not trigger an additional stress response. She could also look at taking five minutes here and there throughout

Table 7.5	Example of action stage dialogue
	Action dialogue
Client:	I'm so tired, I don't feel like training.
Trainer:	Well, you are here and that's a good start, so well done. We can start gently and look at this a little more.
Client:	OK. (*reluctantly*)
Trainer:	(*During warm-up*) How are you feeling?
Client:	I still feel tired. I know I will feel better once I've done it, it's just getting here.
Trainer:	Well, you got here and we've started and that's great. We can look at some other ways of helping you to maintain your energy through the day. Your tiredness could be related to what you are eating or drinking through the day. Maybe you could also treat yourself to a soak in the jacuzzi at the end of this to massage away some of the extra tension?
Client:	Oh, yes, that's a nice thought.
Trainer:	It's also a little reward to yourself for getting here and making the effort and that is important.

the day to complete some desk exercises that can help reduce muscle tension. These possibilities provide an alternative response to the stimulus or trigger (counter-conditioning), a strategy that can help to manage stress more positively. It is also useful to have a contingency plan to help the client maintain motivation when she or he feels tempted to relapse. See table 7.5 for a sample action stage dialogue.

Maintenance

At this stage of the change process the individual is sustaining the changes and preventing relapse. The new habit may be established and some coping strategies will be in place for managing problem situations and avoiding temptation.

The role of the personal trainer at this stage is to provide a helpful and supportive relationship and reinforce the positive behaviour by giving plenty of praise and encouragement, which acts as a reward and can help to increase the client's self-efficacy. The client will also need reminding of all the successes to help maintain motivation. He or she will also need to be made aware of possible cues that may indicate the likelihood of a relapse and have strategies in place to manage a relapse. It may be worthwhile to educate the client on how thought processes may respond in times of relapse. Some clients will *overgeneralise* and see the slip as meaning a complete failure. Others may experience *selective abstraction* where they focus only on the failure and not on any of the successes. Other clients will take *excessive responsibility* for the slip and see it as their own personal weakness. Others will *catastrophise* and go totally overboard and exaggerate how bad the slip was. Some clients use a mixture or even all of these thought processes to throw themselves out of the change cycle. It is useful if the trainer can work with the client to help them recognise where potential slips may be attributed. For example, a client who sees a slip as his own lack of willpower will experience a reduction in self-efficacy and personal power if he relapses, whereas a client who believes a slip is just a temporary lack of coping will maintain self-efficacy and is more likely to get back into the cycle. It is therefore useful if the trainer works with the client and explains that slips are often a natural occurrence until a new habit or change of behaviour is imprinted. It is worth recognising that even changing the way they think is a challenge for most people. For example, if we have spent 30–40 years thinking self-critical or negative thoughts, then it will be a big challenge to break that behaviour pattern. A client who has smoked for 20 years will have an equal challenge to break a number of behaviour patterns that include buying cigarettes, lighting them, the hand-to-mouth action, the inhaling and so on. There are many behaviours that would have to change and each step the client makes is a success! It is essential to highlight all of these. See table 7.6 for a sample maintenance stage dialogue.

Relapse

At this stage of the cycle of change the client would have returned to their old behaviour. For example,

Table 7.6	Example of dialogue to maintain change and manage relapse
	Maintenance/relapse dialogue
Client:	I'm a failure. We went out for a meal yesterday and I ate loads. I had XX for starters and XX for a main course and then XX for dessert and I had cheese and biscuits as well (*looks sheepish*) and two Irish coffees with cream.
Trainer:	How does that feel?
Client:	It makes me think I'm a failure and I feel I let myself down.
Trainer:	So when you think you have failed you feel like you've let yourself down?
Client:	Yeah... (*looks thoughtful*)
Trainer:	So you have kept to your exercise programme regularly and you've been eating sensibly for three months and the first time you go out for a meal and you pig out, you are a failure?
Client:	Well, that's how it feels.
Trainer:	What makes you think you have failed?
Client:	Well, today I thought 'You ate all that yesterday, you might as well just give up.'
Trainer:	Well, you are training again today, that's another positive action. If you feel that bad, you could always start using your food diary again and notice the thoughts and feelings around when you are tempted to go off track and you can use some positive thinking strategies to help you. Maybe you just need to be a little easier on yourself? You have managed the change for a long time, one slip when you were in a very tempting situation can be allowed, surely?

they may have stopped exercising, or returned to old eating or lifestyle patterns. Relapse is an uncomfortable experience as it increases feelings of failure and hopelessness, which discourages the client and makes her or him lose confidence and the belief in her or his ability to make changes.

At this stage the trainer can give support and encouragement and explore possible causes for the relapse, then review the client's action plan and work with the client to help him or her re-enter the change cycle.

Termination

The new behaviour would be permanent at this stage, and the goal achieved.

It usually takes clients a few attempts to move through the change cycle and a few relapses are experienced before they get to this stage. The change process in reality is not so orderly, people get stuck at specific stages a few times before they move towards changing behaviours and habits permanently.

The model represents the different levels of psychological functioning that interrelate and that require work to help the person make the desired changes. These are:

- presenting problem (the behaviour)
- negative thought processes (thinking)
- interpersonal difficulties (relationship with others)

Table 7.7	Example of dialogue to manage total relapse
	Relapse dialogue
Client:	I feel really depressed. All the good things I was going to do to help manage my stress have just gone out of the window and it just seems pointless.
Trainer:	Oh, that sounds like it is really awful for you.
Client:	Yes, it is. I feel like a complete failure and that all my efforts are wasted.
Trainer:	Maybe you could use this as a learning experience. You made so many positive changes and managed for a long time. Maybe seeing it all go out of the window is also a positive. At least you know a little more about what causes you to give up on it all and maybe you needed to for a while?
Client:	Maybe...
Trainer:	Well, you can start bringing in small changes again anytime you want to, it only has to be one small step at a time.
Client:	I guess so...
Trainer:	How about you start really simply and just work on some positive thinking to boost how you feel about yourself for a starter, you deserve that!
Client:	Yes, and I guess that might make me feel a little bit more confident about making other changes?
Trainer:	Absolutely, one step at a time.

- social/systemic difficulties (relationship with systems)
- intrapersonal difficulties (relationship with self).

Personal trainers can recognise where the person is within the cycle of change and this will help them to identify appropriate interventions they are qualified to manage, and also where their expertise ends and additional professional support, such as counselling, may be needed.

Personal trainers can help with the behavioural and, to some extent, the thinking levels of functioning. They would not be professionally qualified to deal with interpersonal, social or intrapersonal conflicts or difficulties the person may be experiencing. This highlights the importance of working with other professionals in a multidiscipline team to manage the change process effectively. Contacts for sources of further help are provided at the end of this book.

A strategic approach towards taking action to change

Making the decision to change certain aspects of one's lifestyle is a positive step, but sometimes the changes themselves can feel a little uncomfortable and provide initial stress. The key to any successful change is to take one step at a time and learn from the experience.

The following 10 steps can be used as a list of strategies to assist with managing any change (reducing stress, increasing activity, changing lifestyle habits and eating patterns).

1. Make a list of all the things that you would like to change.
2. Decide what changes are the most important to you.
3. Raise your awareness of the advantages and disadvantages of changing each behaviour and aspect.
4. Work out specific goals for each aspect to create the change you desire.

5. Get to know more about each behaviour and the things you want to change by keeping a diary.
6. Identify what alternative strategies and behaviours you could use when your behaviour is triggered.
7. Prepare to make the changes.
8. Set the date where you will start making changes.
9. Be ready to cope with setbacks.
10. Stay motivated – get support!

Step 1: Make a list of all the things that you would like to change

The things people would like to change in their life will vary from individual to individual. Most people would like to make some changes. These may include:

- changing jobs
- taking a study course
- moving abroad
- taking more exercise
- lowering stress levels
- giving up smoking
- drinking less alcohol
- reducing fat in your diet
- eating more vegetables.

Step 2: Decide what changes are the most important to you

Prioritise the things you would like to change and select what seems to be the most appropriate thing for you to start with. Some people will need to make changes that offer specific results (for example losing weight). Other people like to succeed at managing the easier changes, which boosts their confidence to make the more difficult ones. Some people like to tackle the toughest change straight away. The key is finding the right way for yourself.

Step 3: Raise your awareness of the advantages and disadvantages of changing a particular behaviour

Use the decisional balance sheet on page 110 to work out the advantages and disadvantages, as these will ultimately identify factors that will affect your commitment to the change process. It will also help you to identify specific blocks.

Identifing blocks

Take a blank piece of paper and draw a pathway.
Write your goal at some point along the path.
Draw closed gates to indicate all the blocks that may prevent you from being successful.
A block could be a person, an occasion, a feeling, a thought process and so on.
Take some time to think of ways that you can open these gates.
Use the exercises listed in Part Two to help you find ways to open the gates and maintain commitment to the change process.

Step 4: Work out specific goals for creating the change you desire

Use the SMART method. Make your goals:

Specific – decide what you want.
Measurable – how will you know you are succeeding?
Achievable – is your goal possible?
Reward yourself – treat yourself as you achieve.
Time-framed – set time limits for goals.

Step 5: Get to know more about your behaviour and the things you want to change by keeping a diary

Before making any changes, get to know your behaviour more. You can record thoughts, feelings, environment (where you are and who you are with) and what triggers the behaviour and so on. You can use the behaviour change diary provided.

The key is to record the following:

Example	Antecedent	Behaviour	Consequence
Eating	Someone upsets you, you feel alone and fed up	Eat biscuits	Feel more cheerful
Smoking	You get stuck in traffic	Light up a cigarette	Feel more relaxed
Drinking	You get home from work tired	Have a glass of wine	Feel de-stressed

Behaviour change diary	Antecedent	Behaviour	Consequence
11a.m.	Felt frustrated Was worrying about...	Had a cigarette Ate biscuits	Felt relieved Felt comforted
Morning			
Afternoon			
Evening			

- Antecedents – what happens before the behaviour.
- Behaviour – what you want to change.
- Consequences – how you felt afterwards.

Step 6: Identify what alternative strategies you could you use when your behaviour is triggered

Use the problem-solving sheet to identify both proactive and reactive strategies for coping.

Problem-solving sheet

What is the specific problem?

What are possible solutions?
(Find as many as possible. You can ask friends or others to contribute their possible solutions.)

Test the solutions
(Be your own experimenter, try different things.)

Evaluate the results
(Find out what works for you and what doesn't and explore the reasons. Find out more about yourself and your behaviour.)

Repeat the process

NB: Sometimes it is necessary to try out a few possible solutions to identify what works and what doesn't work and learn from the experience. There are always other solutions.

Some proactive (thinking ahead) strategies are:

Problem: Eating because you feel alone or fed up

- Phone a friend and talk, share your feelings.
- Go for a walk.
- Join a group activity.
- Eat a healthy snack.

Problem: Smoking when stuck in traffic

- Have fruit or raw vegetables or mints in the car instead of cigarette.
- Put your cigarettes out of reach.
- Create the routine of taking deep breaths when in traffic.

Problem: Having a drink to relax immediately on arriving home

- Go to the gym before going home.
- Plan a course of relaxation exercises before you sit down and have a drink.
- Go for a walk before you have a drink.
- Drink a glass of water first.

Problem: As you are ready to leave work your boss gives you some extra work

- Attend an assertiveness course and negotiate with your boss about an appropriate time for giving additional work.
- Look around for another job.

Reactive strategies (thinking on your feet) are required when the behaviour is triggered unexpectedly. The positive aspect of this is that the more you have experimented with different ways of changing, the more you learn and the more reactive strategies you may potentially have available.

Some examples are:
- taking some deep breaths
- using positive self-talk
- removing yourself from the situation at a specific time and going for a walk
- drawing a picture
- talking to a friend to manage the feelings.

When certain feelings are triggered it is an automatic response to reach for a known comfort aid or revert to the most known way of coping. This is OK. The key is to learn from the experience of the relapse and get back on that wagon again, believing in yourself and knowing that you *can* do it and that you *can* cause the desired changes to happen. It is committing yourself fully to the process.

Step 7: Prepare to make the changes

Once you have identified what you want to change, what triggers your behaviour and how much you indulge yourself in this behaviour, start to build in small, manageable changes using the following FIT principles:

- Frequency – how often you do the activity
- Intensity – the amount you indulge
- Time – how long you spend doing it.

Table 7.8 gives you some examples

Step 8: Set the date where you will start to make changes

Make the commitment to yourself to change. You can write this commitment down in a journal, share it with a friend, put a sticker on the fridge or use the personal commitment sheet provided. The key is to make sure that whatever you have planned to do must be SMART and

---

Personal commitment

I (print name) have decided:

The things I would like to change are:
I would like to change these because:
The changes I have chosen to make are:
I will make these changes by:
My support network includes:
Some challenges may be:
My coping strategies include:
I will know I have succeeded when:
My reward to myself for succeeding will be:

Signed:

Date:

---

workable for you. Make short-term goals, medium-term goals and long-term goals that help you move towards the change you desire.

Step 9: Be ready to cope with setbacks

It is fairly common for things not to run exactly to plan. It is easier to recover if you are prepared. Take a look at all the problem situations and blocks you have identified and the strategies you decided on to work with these and be ready to enforce them.

Avoid complacency

Missing one exercise session, having one cigarette or having a diet hiccup does not make a difference *unless* it prevents you from starting again. If you slip, aim to recommit to the change.

Beware of high-risk situations

It may be easier to avoid situations initially where friends are drinking alcohol and smoking, for example.

Be assertive

Say 'No thank you' if you are offered a cigarette or cake. Commit to your decision with power rather than saying 'I'd love to, but...'

Coping with craving

Be ready for strong urges that you will want to give in to. They do not last for long but can feel very intense. Be prepared for them and have strategies for dealing with them; for example, call a supportive friend.

Reward yourself

Plan a whole range of small rewards for each success. Use some of the creature comforts suggested in Part Two as a starting point. You

Table 7.8	Applying FIT principles to behaviour		
	Eating	*Drinking*	*Smoking*
Frequency	Eat take-out meals on fewe rdays of the week Have a chocolate-free day	Reduce the number of days you drink or go to the pub Have a drink-free day	Reduce the number of cigarettes you smoke in one day Have a smoke-free day
Intensity	If you eat take-out meals choose a healthier option	Reduce the quantity of alcohol you consume in one go Have drinks with mixers so less alcohol is consumed	Take fewer inhalations of each cigarette Smoke a lighter brand Use a cigarette filter
Time	Eat more slowly Take a break between courses so you allow yourself the experience of feeling full	Go to the pub later in the day	Delay each cigarette by 5–10 min
	Stress when driving	*Negative thinking and self-talk*	*Self-time*
Frequency	Walk instead of driving where possible Use public transport	Take 5 minutes at regular intervals in the day to speak positive affirmations to yourself	Plan regular moments in each day to take some time out for yourself Put specific things in your diary each week that are just for you
Intensity	Listen to a positive-thinking tape as you drive Speak some positive affirmations as you drive	Write the affirmations in a journal and read it regularly Look at yourself in the mirror when you speak your affirmations Stick positive messages and posters around your home and at work as positive reminders	Make each of your self-treats really indulgent (e.g. massage) Choose an activity you really love and haven't done for ages and make time for this
Time	On long journeys stop for regular breaks and read a book or magazine Take some rest intervals in your journey Give yourself extra time to get to places so you feel less harried	Use your affirmations as you walk to work Increase the time you spend on giving yourself positive self-talk	Start with small durations of self-time and increase these gradually

may choose a day at a health spa, a new outfit, a bubble bath, a massage. If you are giving up smoking, save the money you would spend on cigarettes and use it for rewards. If you want to lose weight, buy a new outfit to celebrate your achievements.

Step 10: Stay motivated!

Staying motivated while implementing any new behaviour is a key to successful change. The secret is having the right support systems that can provide you with the help you need to make the changes. These support systems can come from a range of sources:

- family
- friends
- a support group where you can work with like-minded people
- self – by using positive self-talk and encouragment
- a personal trainer
- a counsellor
- a self-help book or seminar.

You can use the grid of life boxes (table 7.9) as a daily diary to record your achievements in each area of your life. Fill each box with one thing you would like to do or that you did to make a difference to each area of your own life. Start noticing the differences you make.

Table 7.9	Life boxes		
Study	Exercise	Friends	Work/career
Relaxation	Personal and spiritual growth	Family	Social
Nutrition	Contribution	Relationship	Home

CREATING A HELPING RELATIONSHIP – INTERPERSONAL SKILLS AND TECHNIQUES TO ASSIST CHANGE 8

Building rapport and relationships

Carl Rogers (1967) listed three primary core conditions for building a positive relationship to bring about successful change. These conditions are: empathy, unconditional positive regard (warmth) and congruency (honesty).

Empathy is the ability to put yourself into the other person's position and see things from his or her perspective. In order to do this we need to be aware of any prejudices and closed-mindedness within us and put these issues to one side. This will help to minimise projection of one's own issues on to the client. It will also help to maximise the communication of positive messages either verbally or non-verbally through our body language. Erskine (2001) proposes the idea of moving beyond empathy by using inquiry skills that enable the person to tell their own story. For example, if a client tells you of a stressful situation, a personally empathic response may be to suggest 'that would make me feel furious'. This type of response can be useful and may help clients contact possibly denied feelings. However, an alternative response would be to ask the client how the stressful situation made him feel. This enables him to use his own voice and describe his own feelings in response to a situation.

Unconditional positive regard is about showing respect and warmth for the person with whom you are working. It is about sending positive messages to them regardless of any judgements you may hold about their behaviour or story. For example, a person who constantly relapses from their intended exercise plan because they are too busy may stir up feelings of frustration. These feelings need to be acknowledged within the self and it may, at some point, be worth inquiring about these feelings. For example, 'How does it make you feel when you miss your exercise programme?' The client may then acknowledge these feelings and the process can be moved on by asking them, 'How can we work together to move through this barrier?' Unconditional positive regard is about accepting the whole person and respecting the self they are presenting as an aspect of the person. It is about accepting their humanness, the difficulties they may experience and the effect these have on their life and self-esteem. It is fairly normal for human beings to dislike and judge certain human behaviours and have prejudices. However, in order to demonstrate unconditional positive regard one needs to be aware of these and take responsibility for these judgements as one's own. These judgements should not be used to condemn or disempower the other person.

Congruency is about being totally honest and communicating and expressing oneself with genuine feeling. It is worth noting that 55 per cent of our communication comes from body language, 38 per cent comes from voice tone and 7 per cent comes from the words we use. Clearly, any discrepancy between what we say and how we feel will be communicated.

The response we get from our communication may actually tell us more about what we are communicating than what we say, or how we say it. In the example above, with the client who relapses from his exercise plan, to deny or ignore your feeling of frustration may be to miss gathering some key information about what the client may be feeling about himself. Awareness of one's own internal processes can enable more effective inquiry about the client's experience.

Rogers (1967) believed that applying these core conditions to a helping relationship would facilitate the person to develop a strong enough sense of self to move forward and make changes.

As personal trainers we need to recognise that while we have certain pieces of knowledge the client needs, it is the client who knows her or his lifestyle and what changes will work in her or his life. Resistance to our 'useful' suggestions should be acknowledged as an indicator that somehow this advice is not right for this client. A more effective approach than giving specific advice such as 'do this' and 'do that' is to offer a range of potential ways for clients to make the changes they desire and allow them to choose which works for them.

Gathering information

Prior to devising an exercise and stress management programme we need to find out about the client's lifestyle. The information we need includes:

- personal details of the client (name, age, address)
- medical health history
- lifestyle information (work, habits, stress levels)
- medication (what type, how long taken for, any recent changes?)

- previous exercise experience
- current exercise and activity levels
- expectations and goals
- likes and dislikes
- any positive strategies that are already in place
- barriers to making changes
- personal motivation and desire to make changes
- support systems to assist with the change process
- what stressors are present in her or his life?
- what coping strategies are currently being used and are these positive or negative?
- what is the client's current mental attitude about his or her life and about making changes?
- how does the client manage emotions?

Motivational interviewing

Motivational interviewing is a client-centred method of gathering information to explore a client's readiness to change. It can be used to elicit information about the client's concerns about specific areas of their life that they would like to change. This information can be then be used to discuss with the person the advantages and disadvantages of making the changes they propose. The information collected can also indicate where the client is in relation to the cycle of change model (contemplating, preparing, action) and can identify their personal levels of motivation, the support system they have in place and any resistance or ambivalence to making changes. It can also help the personal trainer to provide the appropriate support and intervention to help the client make a positive decision for herself. Finally, it enables the personal trainer to negotiate goals and strategies to work towards with their client.

Questioning

Asking questions can be an effective method for gathering initial and further information from the client. However, there can sometimes be a tendency to ask too many questions, which may block some clients from speaking if they feel they are under interrogation. It may also prevent us from listening effectively and actively to what the client is saying.

Personal trainers tend to use questioning to gather factual information from their clients. This is essential for some information; however, sometimes it is necessary to use questioning also as a form of inquiry to gain a fuller picture of the person's subjective experience.

There are different types of questions: **open questions** are questions that begin with the words What? Who? How? Where? Why? When? and are most effective for gathering information in greater depth. These types of question will generally enable the client to relax and will encourage them to speak openly. For example, 'How did you feel when you were faced with that confrontation at work?' 'How did you feel when you broke from your diet?' 'Would you like to explore that further?'

Further information can be gathered from open questioning by following up with **probing questions** to encourage the client to expand on their initial response, or with **focusing questions** to enquire more closely about a specific response that may help to define the problem more clearly. For example:

Probing: 'Could you explain that?' 'Tell me more about that?' 'Have you ever experienced that sensation before?'

Focusing: 'Tell me more about the tension you feel in your body when you experience confrontation' 'What do you think that sensation is telling you?' 'Would you like to explore that sensation further?'

Questioning pitfalls

Asking closed questions: for example, 'So that's the reason you felt stressed?' These questions frequently provide only a yes or no or a single response, and close down dialogue. They can also give the impression that the person is not being heard or listened to, which can add to frustration.

Asking multiple questions: For example, 'Have you spoken to your boss about that? or are you scared to approach them? Do you think they will be angry with you?' This style of questioning is confusing because the person will be unsure which one to respond to and this may add to emotional distress.

Asking leading questions: For example, 'Wouldn't you feel better if you did your exercise before you went out to have a drink?' This style of questioning leads the person towards the trainer's way of thinking, and has a judgemental and patronising feel, which can put the person under pressure and add to their frustration.

Interpersonal skills

Focusing on the client

Make the client the most important person in the room and demonstrate this by:

- facing forwards and looking at him or her
- removing any barriers such as desks
- being interested and attentive
- being sensitive to your own facial expressions and body language
- minimising distractions by using a private room, placing a do not disturb sign on the door and ensuring mobile phones are switched off
- leaning forwards slightly, but not so far that you appear aggressive
- keeping an open body and upright posture that is comfortable but not too stiff

- maintaining eye contact without staring
- reflecting warmth by demonstrating the core conditions
- smiling naturally and being present for the client
- avoiding fidgeting.

Listening

Listening and hearing what the client is saying is a real skill and requires practice.

You can demonstrate that you are listening in the following ways:

- Making some acknowledgement when the client is speaking. For example, nodding your head or saying 'yes'.
- Summarising what you have heard the client say in your own words, telling them what you think you have heard them say and allowing them to correct you. For example, 'Am I hearing you say that you feel ... when this happens?'
- Reflecting back what the client says. For example, 'So when you miss your exercise programme you get frustrated with yourself and this makes you feel worse.'
- Asking questions if you do not understand or if you need further information than what the client is saying. For example, 'Would you tell me more about that so I can get a better picture?'

> 'Do you listen with the same enthusiasm with which you speak?'
>
> Richard Wilkins

Recognising your own barriers to listening effectively

There are a number of barriers that can stop us from listening effectively; some of these include:

Relating everything to yourself and your own experience. For example, 'Yes, I find it difficult to make time to relax as well.' This may be true, but it is not useful for helping your client explore their barriers to making the change.

Thinking about the next question you want to ask your client. If you are spending time thinking about your next question, you are not listening to what they are saying. You may also be switching off to some vital information they are giving you.

Switching off and letting your mind daydream. If this happens it is more respectful to apologise, acknowledge this and ask the client to repeat what they were saying.

Making internal judgements on what the client has said. Judging your client as unmotivated, lazy or any other judgement you make internally will block you from listening to what the client is saying and also block your ability to be able to offer help.

Interrupting and giving advice. For example, if the client says she struggles to find time to relax, don't tell her what she should do to make time. It is more helpful to suggest to the client that maybe you could both explore different ways that would help her to manage her time.

Ignoring expressions of emotion with shallow, unempathic comments such as, 'Well, it could be worse.' These are unhelpful in that they draw attention away from what the client is experiencing. Exploration of these emotions can be crucial to identifying ways for them to move forward and make positive changes.

Other blocks to listening may include:

- tiredness
- personal stress and problems
- personal differences (culture, gender, age)
- having experiences similar to those of the client
- not being able to relate to the client's experience.

CASE STUDIES

PART **FOUR**

4

This section explores specific case studies and the techniques used to exercise away the subject's stress. The case studies include:

Case study 1: Single, 35-year-old, apparently healthy female. Employed full-time.

Case study 2: Married, 59-year-old female with mild depression, osteoporosis and osteo-arthritis. Employed full-time. Two grown-up children (one dependent due to disability).

Case study 3: Married (to case study 4), 46-year-old female with hypothyroidism and mild stress. Runs family business with partner. Two children (one teenager living at home).

Case study 4: Married (to case study 3), 50-year-old male, overweight, inactive, with mild stress. Runs family business with partner. Two children (one teenager living at home).

Case study 5: Married, 39-year-old female, apparently healthy. Mother to four children and full-time carer (with some assistance) for disabled son. Voluntary counselling work two days per week.

As a starting point for working with clients experiencing stress, the following areas are provided as directions for gathering information and working with the client:

- current activity levels
- fitness goals and health status
- current stressors
- support systems
- positive and negative coping strategies
- relaxation time
- how stress manifests (physical, behavioural, mental and emotional)
- possible strategies identified by client and trainer.

The techniques suggested and programmed to assist with managing stress at a mental, emotional, physical and behavioural level are those explained throughout Part Two of this book.

There is also a list of some quick-fix strategies for different time-frames and different scenarios listed at the end of this section.

CASE STUDIES

Case study 1

- Female, 35, white, single, no children.
- Full time employee – stressful job, long hours at desk with two hours travelling per day.
- Lives alone, own home – mortgaged.

Currently activity levels	Attends exercise class for 1 hour on 2–3 days per week. Walks for ½ hour with friend 2 days a week. Walks to and from station every day. Walks to shops and whenever she can.
Fitness goals	Would like to improve cardiovascular fitness but limited time at the moment. Would like to improve muscle tone/definition by working out in gym, but has limited time at the moment.
Health status	Apparently healthy. Some stress.
Current stressors	Work pressures: some role confusion, lack of support, feels pulled in all directions. Long hours. Travelling. Financial difficulties. Limited disposable income.
Support systems	Supportive circle of friends.
Positive coping strategies	Regular exercise and activity. Speaks with friends. Takes some time out to relax and for creature comforts. Visits counsellor every two weeks.
Negative coping resources	Smoking – this increases when feeling overwhelmed. Alcohol – drinks most evenings to unwind. Diet – is aware of need to eat more regularly and eat healthier foods. Tends to eat ready meals that are easy to cook.
Relaxation time	Has free time some evenings and weekends free. In evenings tends to feel tired and wants to just cosy up, especially in winter. Weekends – occasional social activities and fun with friends. Tends to use weekends to complete college assignments for part-time study course.

Signs and symptoms of stress

Mental signs and symptoms indicated	
Irrational thoughts	Occasionally
Poor decision-making	Occasionally
Low self-worth	Occasionally
Procrastination	Yes
Ego-centred	Occasionally

Emotional signs and symptoms indicated	
Angry	Occasionally
Scared/fearful	Yes
Bored	Yes
Lonely	Yes
Powerless	Occasionally
Insecure	Occasionally
Frustrated	Yes
Lethargic	Yes
Unfocused	Occasionally
Tearful	Occasionally
Anxious	Yes

Physical signs and symptoms indicated	
Spots	Yes
Shoulder tension	Occasionally
Clenched jaw	Occasionally

Behavioural signs and symptoms indicated	
Drinking more stimulants	Yes
Smoking more	Yes
Crying	Yes
Picking at skin	Yes
Exercising more or less	Yes

Possible strategies identified by case study 1 and trainer

Physical and behavioural	Visit GP for medication for skin irritation and spots. Decrease smoking and drink less caffeine. Massage to release muscle tension. Eat more vegetables, cereal, fruit and fibre type foods. Add one gym session to training programme with personal trainer. 5 minutes desk exercises to release muscle tension at work. Work towards finding alternative strategies to manage smoking (smoking cessation) and drinking (plan to have 2–3 alcohol-free days). Start weekend mornings with a walk or a visit to the gym. Find a training buddy for gym work. Plan meals ahead, write a list before shopping. Keep a diary to record how lifestyle behaviours are affected by stress and emotions. 5 min yoga (2 postures in the morning) some mornings.
Mental and emotional	Regular positive affirmations, especially during stressful times, to maintain self-efficacy. Can buy or record own positive affirmation tapes to play while travelling by train to and from work. Read self-help book while travelling. Be own best friend and affirm ability to handle situations. Deep breathing to calm panic. Share fear and upset feelings with supportive friends and allow support. Pent-up anger, frustration and confusion can be managed by exercise or creative work. Find more time to socialise and have fun.

Strategies selected by case study 1:

- Reduce coffee intake.
- Include one personal training exercise session per week.
- Plan social activities at least once a week.
- Perform desk exercises (5 minutes each day).
- Prepare healthier food and drink more water.
- Play relaxation tape on way home from work and take self-help book for journey to work.
- Book one body massage a month.
- Do some creative drawing and writing to release emotions.

Weekly log for case study 1

Day/date	6am–10am	10am–2pm	2pm–6pm	6pm onwards
Monday	Walk to station **Relaxation tape on train**	**Desk mobility exercises**	**Relaxation tape on way home**	Walk from station **Exercise class**
Tuesday	Walk to station		**Relaxation and breathing work 5 minutes**	Walk from station Relaxing evening **Creative drawing**
Wednesday	Walk to station **Relaxation tape on train**	**Desk mobility exercises**		Walk from station Go walking with friend
Thursday	Walk to station **Read self-help book on train**			Walk from station Exercise class
Friday	Walk to station **Read self-help book on train**	**Desk mobility exercises**	**Relaxation tape on way home**	Walk from station
Saturday		**Personal training gym session with steam room and jacuzzi afterwards** Plan and complete weekly shop	Study time	**Social**
Sunday	Relax and read magazines	Clean house	Walk in park with friend	

NB: **Bold type indicates newly introduced interventions.**

Case study 2

- Female, 59, white, married, two grown-up children. One child still living at home.
- Full-time employee – stressful job.
- Lives with husband and one child.
- Own home – mortgaged.

Current activity levels	Yoga one day a week. Swimming one day a week.
Fitness goals	To have a little more energy. To improve posture. To reduce joint discomfort.
Health status	Mild osteoporosis and osteo-arthritis. Mild depression. No medication.
Current stressors	Works long hours. Has demanding boss. Doesn't like saying no. Lacks confidence in ability at work. Has to meet family demands. No time for self.
Support systems	No friendship support systems.
Positive coping strategies	Exercises twice a week. Has considered visiting a counsellor.
Negative coping resources	Negative thinking patterns which lower self-esteem. Passive behaviour.
Relaxation time	Has free time in evenings, but feels tired. Has weekends free.

Signs and symptoms of stress

Mental signs and symptoms indicated	
Irrational thoughts	Occasionally
Poor decision-making	Yes
Low self-esteem	Yes
Low self-worth	Yes
Procrastination	Yes
Excessive self-criticism	Yes
Emotional signs and symptoms indicated	
Sad	Yes
Angry	Occasionally
Depressed	Yes
Resentful	Yes
Powerless	Yes
Frustrated	Yes
Unfocused	Yes
Tearful	Yes
Loses hope	Occasionally
Physical signs and symptoms indicated	
Shoulder tension	Yes
Upper back hunched	Yes
Tense forehead/headaches	Yes
Behavioural signs and symptoms indicated	
Crying	Yes

Possible strategies identified by case study 2 and trainer

Physical and behavioural	Explore option of HRT with GP. Massage on a regular basis to release muscle tension. Add walking to weekly activities. Desk exercises to release muscle tension and improve joint mobility. Pilates class to improve posture (and social). 10 minutes yoga in the mornings to help relax and start day positively.
Mental and emotional	Regular meditation to raise awareness of negative thinking. Buy or record own positive affirmation tape to play while driving to and from work. Replace use of words 'ought' and 'should' with 'could'. Attend assertive communication course. Speak with counsellor. Find time for comfort activities for self.
Social	Join other groups/classes: positive thinking and so on.

Strategies selected by case study 2

- Plan one enjoyable social activity with family once a week.
- Perform desk mobility exercises at work.
- Attend assertiveness training course.
- Use positive affirmation tape while travelling to and from work.
- Arrange regular body message and visit to beauty therapist.
- Speak with counsellor to manage feelings of depression.
- Join Pilates class to work on posture.

Weekly log for case study 2

Day/date	6am–10am	10am–2pm	2pm–6pm	6pm onwards
Monday	Positive affirmation tape while driving to work		Desk exercises after lunch	Yoga class
Tuesday	10 minutes yoga with relaxation tape	Walk in lunch hour in local park		Assertiveness course for 10 weeks
Wednesday	10 minutes yoga with relaxation tape		Desk exercises after lunch	Comfort activity for self
Thursday	Positive affirmation tape while driving to work			Swimming Plan family social event
Friday	Positive affirmation tape while driving to work	Walk in lunch hour in local park	Counselling with meditation skills	Comfort activity for self
Saturday		Study course		Plan family social event
Sunday		Pilates class		

NB: Bold type indicates newly introduced interventions.

Case study 3

- Female, 45, married, two children (one teenager).
- Works full-time in family business.
- Lives with husband and one child.
- Own home – mortgaged.

Current activity levels	One personal training session per week. One dance class per week.
Fitness goals	To improve fitness. To lose weight.
Health status	Family history of CHD (coronary heart disease). Hyperthyroidism. Mild arthritis. Stress.
Current stressors	Not sleeping well. Using sleeping tablets. Taking on too much and not saying no. Being overweight adds to stress. Family demands (elderly mother). Work problems. Financial juggling. Not being able to relax. Not making time or finding discipline to exercise regularly.
Support systems	Husband. Good circle of friends. Personal trainer. Regular meals out with friends for social.
Positive coping strategies	Exercise and dance twice a week.
Negative coping resources	Eating more when stressed. Sleeping tablets. Thinks she has no willpower or ability to discipline self.
Relaxation time	Has to make diary commitment to stick to plans and make time for self. Gets distracted easily to do other jobs.

Signs and symptoms of stress

Mental signs and symptoms indicated	
Irrational thoughts	Yes
Mental fatigue	Yes
Poor decision-making	Yes
Low self-esteem	Yes
Low self-worth	Yes
Inability to listen	Yes
Excessive self-criticism	Yes
Emotional signs and symptoms indicated	
Sad	Occasionally
Frustrated	Yes
Tearful	Yes
Physical signs and symptoms indicated	
Inability to sleep	Yes
Dizziness	Occasionally
Behavioural signs and symptoms indicated	
Eating more or less	Yes
Drinking more stimulants	Yes
Crying	Yes
Increased or decreased sexual libido	Yes
Excessive talking	Yes

Possible strategies identified by case study 3 and trainer

Physical and behavioural	Keep food diary to monitor thinking, moods and eating patterns. Plan weekly shop and buy healthier food options (increase vegetables, fruit, jacket potatoes, fish) Eat healthier options when eating out. Drink more water. Plan another exercise session each week (personal training). Plan dance practice with husband on two evenings per week. Attend an assertiveness training course. Add vigour to house cleaning. Decrease coffee (replace with herbal tea).
Mental and emotional	Plan a creature comfort on two days per week. Write a hassle list. Write out thoughts and feelings before going to bed. Have a notepad beside bed for writing down thoughts that interrupt sleep. Play a relaxation tape before going to sleep. Plan a worry hour where you write out all the things that are bothering you. Use house cleaning strategies to manage other problems (one thing at a time). Positive affirmation tape when driving.

Strategies selected by case study 3

- Keep food diary to monitor thinking, moods and eating patterns.
- Plan weekly shop and buy healthier food options (increase vegetables, fruit, jacket potatoes, fish).
- Drink more water.
- Plan dance practice with husband on two evenings per week.
- Plan a creature comfort on two days per week.
- Write a hassle list and plan worry time.
- Have a notepad beside bed for writing down thoughts that interrupt sleep.
- Play a relaxation tape before going to sleep.
- Listen to positive affirmation tape when driving.

Weekly log for case study 3

Day/date	6am–10am	10am–2pm	2pm–6pm	6pm onwards
Monday	Clean house with vigour Worry time and plan week ahead			Relaxation tape before bed
Tuesday	Clean house		Dance practice with partner	Social Relaxation tape before bed
Wednesday	Clean house with vigour	Personal training session		Creature comfort Relaxation tape before bed
Thursday	Clean house		Dance practice with partner	Social Relaxation tape before bed
Friday	Clean house with vigour	Additional exercise session (personal trainer optional)		Creature comfort Relaxation tape before bed
Saturday	Plan family shop	Dance class with partner		Family social
Sunday		Family lunch		

NB: Bold type indicates newly introduced interventions.

Case study 4

- Male, 50, married, two children (one teenager).
- Works full-time in family business.
- Lives with wife and one child.
- Own home – mortgaged.

Current activity levels	One dance class per week with wife.
Fitness goals	Does not feel motivated to exercise at present. Would like to practise dancing.
Health status	Family history of CHD (coronary heart desease). Stress.
Current stressors	Work. People.
Support systems	Wife.
Positive coping strategies	Counsellor. Reads self-help books and makes time for personal development.
Negative coping resources	Drinks more when stressed.
Relaxation time	Makes time to read. Tends to procrastinate when there is time to do things.

Signs and symptoms of stress

Mental signs and symptoms indicated	
Irrational thoughts	Yes
Poor decision-making	Yes
Inability to listen	Yes
Accident proneness	Yes
Making more mistakes	Yes
Emotional signs and symptoms indicated	
Depression	Yes
Jealousy	Yes
Insecurity	Yes
Frustration	Yes
Anxiety	Yes
Physical signs and symptoms indicated	
Nervous indigestion	Yes
Yawning or sighing a lot	Yes
Tense forehead/headaches	Yes
Behavioural signs and symptoms indicated	
Eating more or less	Yes
Drinking more stimulants	Yes
Argumentative, aggressive behaviour (violence or crime)	Yes
Cannot sit still	Yes
Nervous laughter	Yes
Driving faster	Yes

Possible strategies identified by case study 4 and trainer

Physical and behavioural	Plan dance practice for 30 minutes on two evenings per week. Cut down on alcohol, keep a diary to record thoughts, mood and drinking and eating patterns. Choose healthier options when eating out. Go walking with partner. Reduce coffee intake (drink peppermint tea). Drink more water.
Mental and emotional	Use positive affirmation tape when driving. Plan worry time.

Strategies selected by case study 4

- Plan dance practice for 30 minutes on two evenings per week.
- Cut down on alcohol, keep a diary to record thoughts, mood and drinking and eating patterns.
- Go walking with partner.
- Drink more water.
- Use positive affvirmation tape when driving.
- Plan worry time.

Weekly log for case study 4

Day/date	6am–10am	10am–2pm	2pm–6pm	6pm onwards
Monday	**Worry time and plan week ahead with partner**			**Diary to record mood and thoughts**
Tuesday			**Dance practice with partner**	Social
Wednesday				**Diary to record mood and thoughts**
Thursday			**Dance practice with partner**	Social
Friday		**Walk with partner**		**Diary to record mood and thoughts**
Saturday		Dance class with partner		Family social
Sunday		Family lunch		

NB: Bold type indicates newly introduced interventions.

Case study 5

- Female, 38, married, four children (one disabled).
- Works as volunteer counsellor two days per week and study course one day per week. Carer for disabled son.
- Lives with husband and children.
- Own home – mortgaged.

Current activity levels	None at present. Feels always on the go.
Fitness goals	Would like to find time to exercise. Used to walk with friend and go to yoga, but cannot make time for one-hour sessions.
Health status	Minor knee aches (not diagnosed condition) experienced with too much impact or bending work. Stress.
Current stressors	Family demands and caring for disabled son. Study course.
Support systems	Husband. Friends. Therapist/counsellor.
Positive coping strategies	Counsellor/therapist. Speaks with husband and friends. Assertive. Is able to build self-esteem with resources such as positive self-talk.
Negative coping resources	Negative thinking. Eating quick foods (biscuits) and drinking lots of tea.
Relaxation time	Makes time to study. Limited time for self.

Signs and symptoms of stress

Mental signs and symptoms indicated	
Irrational thoughts	Occasionally
Mental fatigue	Occasionally
Poor decision-making	Occasionally
Low self-esteem	Yes
Low self-worth	Yes
Inability to listen	Occasionally
Excessive self-criticism	Yes
Making more mistakes	Yes

Emotional signs and symptoms indicated	
Sad	Yes
Angry	Yes
Scared/fearful	Yes
Panicky	Yes
Irritable	Yes
Lonely	Yes
Resentful	Occasionally
Helpless	Occasionally

Emotional signs and symptoms indicated cont.	
Powerless	Occasionally
Insecure	Occasionally
Frustrated	Yes
Lethargic	Yes
Tearful	Yes
Anxious	Yes
Loses hope	Yes

Physical signs and symptoms indicated	
Spots	Occasionally

Behavioural signs and symptoms indicated	
Eating more or less	Yes
Argumentative, aggressive behaviour (violence or crime)	Occasionally
Crying	Yes
Increased or decreased sexual libido	Yes
Driving faster	Yes

Possible strategies identified by case study 5 and trainer

Physical and behavioural	Plan weekly shop and buy healthier options than quick food (fruit and vegetables, jacket potatoes). Start walking with friend once a week. 5–10 minutes yoga on two days per week. Reduce tea intake (drink peppermint tea). Drink more water. Plan family swim at weekend. Walk kids to school. Plan creature comforts for self.
Mental and emotional	Positive affirmation tape when driving. Plan time management activities (study time, exercise time and so on).

Strategies selected by case study 5

- Go walking with friend.
- Walk kids to school if not raining.
- Do yoga for 10 minutes two mornings a week.
- Drink more water.
- Listen to positive affirmation tape when driving.
- Use time management strategies.
- Plan weekly shop.

Weekly log for case study 5

Day/date	6am–10am	10am–2pm	2pm–6pm	6pm onwards
Monday	**Walk kids to school**	Volunteer	**Positive tape when driving**	Family activities **Creature comfort**
Tuesday	Clean house with vigour		**Walk with friend**	Family activities
Wednesday	10 minutes yoga		Positive affirmation tape when driving	Family activities
Thursday	10 minutes yoga Clean house with vigour	Study course	Study course	Study course
Friday	**Walk kids to school**		Positive affirmation tape when driving	Family activities **Creature comfort**
Saturday		Family activities	Family activities	
Sunday		Family activities	Family activities	**Prepare and plan time for week ahead Plan weekly shop**

NB: Bold type indicates newly introduced interventions.

Summary of quick tips to manage stress

Five-minute strategies

- Posture awareness exercises.
- Breathing exercises.
- Desk mobility exercises.
- Smiling and laughter.
- Positive self-talk.
- Meditation.
- Say no.
- Say yes.

15-minute strategies

- Physical activity (e.g. walking).
- Creative work.
- Creature comforts (some of list).
- Hassles and possibility lists.

30-minute strategies

- Relaxation scripts.
- Physical activity.
- Creative work.
- Creature comforts (some of list).
- Physical fitness and exercise programmes.
- Reading self-help books.
- Listening to self-help motivation tape.
- Worry time.

Techniques when travelling and waiting in queues

- Shoulder mobility from desk exercises.
- Positive affirmation tapes.
- Self-help books.
- Breathing.
- Posture awareness.
- Positive self-talk.
- Letting go.
- Being grateful.

Techniques when driving

- Shoulder mobility from desk exercises.
- Positive affirmation tapes.
- Breathing.
- Posture awareness.
- Letting go and being grateful.

> 'Change and growth take place when a person has risked himself, and dares to become involved in experimenting with his own life'
>
> Herbert Otto

REFERENCES AND RECOMMENDED READING

Axline, V. (1964), *Dibs in Search of Self*, Penguin, London, UK.

Bayne *et al* (1998), *The Counsellor's Handbook*, Stanley Thornes, Cheltenham, UK.

Berne, E. (1964), *Games People Play*, Penguin, London, UK.

Benson, H., MD (1975), *The Relaxation Response*, Avon, New York, USA.

Carlson, R. (1997), *Stop Thinking, Start Living*, Thorsons, London, UK.

Carlson, R. (1998), *The Don't Sweat the Small Stuff Workbook*, Hodder and Stoughton, London, UK.

Erskine, R., Moursand, J. and Troutman, R. (1999), *Beyond Empathy – A Therapy of Contact in Relationships*, Brunner Routledge, New York, USA.

Feltham, C. and Horton, I. (eds) (2000), *Handbook of Counselling and Psychotherapy*, Sage, London, UK.

Forstater, M. and Manuel, J. (2002), *The Spiritual Teachings of Yoga*, Hodder and Stoughton, London, UK.

Fritchie, R. and Melling, M. (1991), *The Business of Assertiveness*, BBC Books, London, UK.

Goleman, D. (1998), *Working with Emotional Intelligence*, Bloomsbury, London, UK.

Gray, J. (1999), *How To Get What You Want and Want What You Have*, Vermilion, London, UK.

Harris, T. (1970), *I'm OK, You're OK*, Pan Books, London, UK.

Hay, L. (1984), *You Can Heal Your Life*, Hay House, Santa Monica, CA, USA.

Haywood, S. and Cohan, M. (1988), *Bag of Jewels*, In-Tune Books, Avalon Beach, NSW, Australia.

Hough, M. (1994), *A Practical Approach to Counselling*, Addison, Wesley, Longman, Harlow, UK.

Hough, M. (1998), *Counselling Skills and Theory*, Hodder and Stoughton, London, UK.

Jeffers, S. (1987), *Feel the Fear and Do It Anyway*, Barnes and Noble, New York, USA.

Jeffers, S. (1996), *End the Struggle and Dance with Life*, Hodder and Stoughton, London, UK.

Jeffers, S. (1998), *Feel the Fear and Beyond*, Rider (Ebury Press), London, UK.

Kobasa, S. (1985), *Conceptualisation and Measurement of Personality in Job Stress Research*, Measures of job stress, NIOSH, New Orleans, USA.

Lawrence, D. (2004), *The Complete Guide to Exercise to Music* (2nd edition), A & C Black, London, UK.

Lawrence, D. (2004), *The Complete Guide to Exercise in Water* (2nd edition), A & C Black, London, UK.

Lindenfield, G. (1989), *Super Confidence*, Thorsons, London, UK.

Looker, T. and Gregson, O. (1997), *Managing Stress*, Hodder and Stoughton, London, UK.

Mcleod, J. (2003), *An Introduction to Counselling*, Open University Press, Milton Keynes, UK.

Phelps, S. and Austin, N. (1997), *The Assertive Woman* (3rd edition), Impact, Atascadero, CA, USA.

Roger, J. and McWilliams, P. (1990), *You Can't Afford the Luxury of a Negative Thought*, Thorsons, London, UK.

Rogers, C. (1967), *On Becoming a Person – A Therapist's View of Psychotherapy*, Constable, London, UK.

Sanders, P. (1996), *First Steps in Counselling* (2nd edition), PCCS Books, Ross on Wye, UK.

Seleye, H. (1956), *The Stress of Life*, McGraw Hill, New York, USA.

Skynner, R. and Cleese, J. (1983), *Families and How to Survive Them*, Vermilion, London, UK.

Steiner, C. (1997), *Achieving Emotional Literacy*, Bloomsbury, London, UK.

TUC (1996), Survey of safety.

Turkington, C. (1998), *Stress Management for Busy People*, McGraw Hill, New York, USA.

Warren, E. and Toll, C. (1993), *The Stress Workbook*, Nicholas Brealey, London, UK.

Wilkins, R. (1998), *Boost Your Life with Mental Tonic*, Cantecia, Northampton, UK.

Wilson, P. (1998), *Calm at Work*, Penguin, London, UK.

USEFUL ADDRESSES

The author
Debbie Lawrence
c/o A & C Black
37 Soho Square
London W1D 3QZ

Personal development workshops, counselling and personal training
For exercise and fitness, stress management, self-esteem, assertiveness, anger management, depression, relaxation and meditation

Exercise and fitness teacher training
YMCA Fitness Industry Training
The Lesley Mowbray Suite
111 Great Russell Street
London WC1B 3NP
www.ymcafit.org.uk

Northern Fitness and Education
9a Cleasby Road
Menston
Ilkley
West Yorkshire LS29 6JE
01943 879816
www.northernfitness.co.uk

Pilates teacher training
Body Control Pilates teacher training
14 Neal's Yard
London WC2 9DP

Pilates Institute and Michael A. King Ltd.
Third floor, Wimbourne House
151–155 New North Road
London N1 6TA

Modern Pilates
www.modernpilates.co.uk
modernpilates@northernfitness.co.uk

Counselling and psychotherapy
BACP (British Association of Counselling and Psychotherapy)
35–37 Albert Street
Rugby CV21 2SG
0870 443 5252
bacp@bacp.co.uk
www.bacp.co.uk

Yoga
Godfrey Devereux
Dynamic Yoga teacher training
36 Stanbridge Road
London SW15 1DX

www.theyogashow.co.uk; www.yogajournal.com; www.sivananda.org; www.yogabasics.com; www.yogafinder.com

Mental health
www.mentalhealth.org.uk; www.anxietycare.org.uk; www.depression.org.uk; www.depressionalliance.org

Stress management
www.stress.org.uk; www.calmcentre.com

Smoking cessation
Quit
102 Gloucester Place
London W1H 3DA

www.stopsmoking.co.uk; www.heartcenteronline.com; www.startquitting.com; www.quitsmoking.com

Alcohol cessation
Alcohol Concern
Waterbridge House
32–36 Loman Street
London SE1 0EE
020 7928 7377
www.alcoholconcern.org.uk

INDEX

W

y